A HEALTHY FUTURE

"*A Healthy Future* presents the deeply human side of the provider caught in the maelstrom of the COVID-19 pandemic as they navigated patient need, political missteps, and their own exhaustion and fear. It is a must-read for anyone who wants to learn the lessons of this dreaded pandemic and build toward a safer and more prepared world."

— Joia Mukherjee, MD, associate professor in global health and social
medicine, Harvard University, and chief medical officer, Partners In Health

"Ryan Meili has extracted the critical lessons of the Saskatchewan COVID-19 experience, highlighting them with his rare combination of humility and courage ... This book is excellent. The lessons are poignant and deeply important."

— Danielle Martin, MD, author of *Better Now: Six Big Ideas to Improve
Healthcare for All Canadians*

"Family doctor and political leader is an unusual combination, but it's one that allows Ryan Meili to deliver a quietly searing diagnosis of how COVID-19 was mishandled in Saskatchewan ... *A Healthy Future* ... provides universal lessons on how to respond to a pandemic and other wrenching socio-political challenges."

— André Picard, author of *Neglected No More: The Urgent Need to
Improve the Lives of Canada's Elders*

"This outstanding book offers a sweeping analysis of this period in recent history: the impact on children, the deadly outbreaks in long-term care facilities, the view from a prison, and many other enlightening perspectives. There are few who witnessed the pandemic from both a seat in the legislature as well as the clinical frontlines of health care, and none who could document it better than this. Meili's honest and frank writing draws out specific lessons and critical messages to which we should pay heed."

— Jane Philpott, former minister of health of Canada, and dean, Faculty
of Health Sciences, Queen's University

"Required reading for anyone who wants to better understand the collective role we all have in ensuring a healthier and more just society."

— Naheed Dosani, MD, palliative care physician and assistant professor,
University of Toronto

"Ryan Meili offers a unique perspective as both a practising politician and a physician. His retelling of the personal impact of the pandemic on so many people reminds us that we were all in it together."

— John Horgan, former premier of British Columbia

"Ryan Meili writes with the compassion of a caring doctor and the passion of a changemaker."

— Raffi Cavoukian, CM, OBC, singer, author, and founder of Child Honouring

"Ryan Meili has a unique vantage point on the COVID-19 pandemic. As both a frontline physician and the leader of the opposition in Saskatchewan, he combines political memoir with pandemic lessons. In a world where we seem eager to revise the past and forget the lessons of COVID-19, Meili provides a clear-eyed view of what happened, what should've happened, and what we can do better next time."

    – Naheed Nenshi, former mayor of Calgary

"If ever anyone can be said to have led the province from the opposition benches, it is Dr. Ryan Meili. His courageous response to the challenge of COVID-19 stood in stark contrast to the lack of leadership from Scott Moe and the Sask Party at a time when it was so desperately needed. That leadership continues with the crystal-clear vision presented in *A Healthy Future.*"

    – Jagmeet Singh, leader of Canada's NDP

"In challenging times, real leaders step up. At the peak of the pandemic, from the halls of the legislature to the halls of the hospital, Ryan Meili did exactly that. *A Healthy Future* is a riveting tale of that challenging time and an important guide to better times ahead."

    – Rachel Notley, former premier of Alberta

"As I read, I kept visualizing the thousands of horror stories from nurses who were trying to do the best they could, even though it was sadly often not enough. This book is an important reminder that a healthy future is not only in the hands of health ministers, just like a strong economy is not only in the hands of finance ministers."

    – Linda Silas, president, Canadian Federation of Nurses Unions

"Canada's prized health care system was under strain long before the COVID pandemic exposed just how vulnerable it is. It's become more important than ever for our elected leaders to refocus on the people that keep our health systems working ... Dr. Ryan Meili offers a clear vision for how Canada and Canadians can push through the status quo, overcoming resistance to change to create a healthier future together.

    – Alika Lafontaine, MD, president, Canadian Medical Association

"*A Healthy Future* is a page-turning account of how the politics of COVID-19 affected provincial responses across Canada. Meili not only identifies issues related to the health care system but ongoing existing problems related to the distribution of economic and social resources ... I will be recommending this book to everyone in my network."

    – Dennis Raphael, author of *Poverty in Canada: Implication for Health and Quality of Life,* and coauthor of *Social Determinants of Health: The Canadian Facts,* 2nd ed.

Ryan Meili

A Healthy Future

Lessons from the Frontlines of a Crisis

PURICH
BOOKS

Purich Books, an imprint of UBC Press
2029 West Mall
Vancouver, BC, V6T 1Z2
www.purichbooks.ca

30 29 28 27 26 25 24 23   5 4 3 2 1

Printed in Canada on FSC-certified ancient-forest-free paper
(100% post-consumer recycled) that is processed chlorine- and acid-free.

Library and Archives Canada Cataloguing in Publication

Title: A healthy future : lessons from the frontlines of a crisis / Ryan Meili.

Names: Meili, Ryan, author.

Description: Includes bibliographical references and index.

Identifiers: Canadiana (print) 20230440363 | Canadiana (ebook) 2023044038X |
ISBN 9780774880909 (softcover) | ISBN 9780774880916 (PDF) |
ISBN 9780774880923 (EPUB)

Subjects: LCSH: COVID-19 Pandemic, 2020—Social aspects—
Saskatchewan. | LCSH: COVID-19 (Disease)—Saskatchewan. |
LCSH: Public health—Saskatchewan.

Classification: LCC RA644.C67 M45 2023 | DDC 362.1962/41440097124—dc23

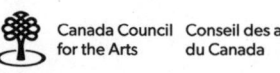 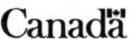

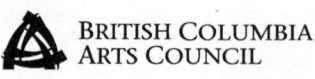 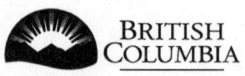

UBC Press gratefully acknowledges the financial support for our publishing
program of the Government of Canada, the Canada Council for the Arts,
and the British Columbia Arts Council.

Unless otherwise indicated, photographs are courtesy of the author.

To my parents, Wally and Lea,
and to Abe and Gus, my little old men

Contents

Foreword
Wisdom in the Scars

Katharine Smart,
past president of the Canadian Medical Association

66

Medicine is a social science, and politics is
nothing more than medicine on a large scale.
– Rudolf Virchow, *Collected Essays*
on Public Health and Epidemiology

In March 2020, I was on holiday with my family for spring break when overnight the world shut down. We started talking about "social distancing," businesses started closing, and we were flooded with new information by the minute. We knew we had to get back home to Whitehorse as soon as possible, so we changed our flights and arrived just hours after the first quarantine rules came into place. I remember sitting on the plane and looking at the people around me wondering if we would all be okay.

My family and I were isolating, and my colleagues and I were scrambling. At the time, I was president of the Yukon Medical Association and had recently been elected to become the 2021–22 president of the Canadian Medical Association. I found myself in hours of meetings as we all worked to figure out what to do and how to make sure care kept flowing to patients. We worked with the government to pivot all our outpatient care to virtual within forty-eight hours. The stress among physicians was palpable as we tried to understand what PPE (personal protective equipment) would be available and how we would potentially manage many very sick people in our tiny hospital thousands of kilometres from anywhere else. We were scared.

Every Canadian's life has been touched by COVID-19. The collective trauma we endured as a nation will have generational impacts. Those impacts are being borne disproportionately by those already marginalized. Workers, people of colour, the elderly, and those living in poverty have carried the burden most intensely, and far too many have died. Children have lost months of education and the normal social interactions of childhood, and many have lost a parent, grandparent, or loved one. Misinformation has cost many Canadians their lives, threatened our social cohesion, and worsened polarization. Previous pandemics have heralded great social change, and I suspect this one will be no different. What will be the legacy of COVID-19? What will we learn? How will we change?

The COVID-19 global pandemic was the first to be fought with the tools of modern science. In Canada, our public health officials warned that ongoing cuts to public health infrastructure would leave us ill prepared and at risk. But the echoes of SARS, MERS, and H1N1 influenza did not reverberate loudly enough for governments to invest adequately in public health funding.

The field of public health was not alone in its state of decline. Canada's beloved "universal" health care system remains neglected. As we move closer to the complete collapse of health care systems across our country – and further away from delivering on the promise of universal health care – patients and providers are suffering. Meanwhile, the inadequate deployment of government resources upstream to create social supports and economic justice has left many Canadians unhealthy. Health is found in a society rooted in principles of equity and justice for all – not inside a hospital or doctor's office.

Advocacy is a core competency of being a physician. For many of us, our desire to advocate for our patients and communities connects us to our purpose in medicine. The pandemic challenged us in new ways to consider what was at stake and what it meant to be an effective advocate. Along with a new and novel virus, we were battling a parallel "infodemic," equally dangerous and spreading just as quickly. Physicians and other health care professionals met this challenge head on by stepping into social and traditional media to share the facts, combat misinformation, and inform the public. This new brand of public-facing advocacy often came with a heavy price.

The impact of the COVID-19 pandemic on health care workers has been profound and unrelenting. We were the early heroes of the pandemic, celebrated around the world with pots and pans and messages of encouragement. As the world locked down, health care workers continued to go to work despite limited access to PPE and concern for their safety and the safety of their families. Some chose to live apart from their families, others changed and showered in their garages, and many wrote wills and made plans for their children while trying to forget about the worst-case scenario.

As Canadians became divided around issues like vaccine mandates and public health protections, our health care system was pushed to its limits. Burnout among health care workers soared. Health care workers went from heroes to the targets of harassment and intimidation – both in person and online. Protests at hospitals, online threats, and escalating violence inside hospitals culminated in the need for federal legislation – Bill C3, which made it illegal to harass or intimidate a health care worker. Later we saw our nation's capital occupied by citizens who did not agree with the public health protections enacted to keep as many Canadians as safe as possible. Throughout, regardless of the risks to themselves and their families, the social upheaval, the harassment, and the trolling, Canada's health care workers continued to show up for Canadians. Today, as we continue to navigate a failing system, these same people are still here caring for others, often at huge personal cost.

In *A Healthy Future: Lessons from the Frontlines of a Crisis*, family doctor and political leader Ryan Meili takes us back to the beginning of the pandemic and walks us through each wave with incredible detail and insight. From his unique position, he reminds us of what we went through and of the political decisions that either saved lives or cost them.

As we moved deeper into the pandemic, science found itself fractured along political lines. Some provinces started to make decisions around public health protections that were based more in politics than science. Several provinces saw their health care systems pushed to the brink and beyond – and both patients and health care workers became the casualties. One such place was my home province of Saskatchewan. During the Delta wave, Saskatchewan had the highest death rate and highest rate of ICU hospitalizations per capita in the country. Physicians across the province organized to publicly call on the government to enact public health measures to protect both citizens and hospitals. In September of 2021, the Canadian Medical Association issued a plea to the governments of Alberta and Saskatchewan to listen to their doctors and take action to save lives.[1] Tragically, those pleas were ignored and the health care system in Saskatchewan was pushed beyond its limits, to the point that by October, ICU patients were being flown to Ontario for care.

What the public couldn't see was the profound moral injury doctors and other health care workers experienced as they tried to persuade the government to act. Many physician leaders were trapped in the dance between their roles, their duty to maintain confidentiality, the expectations put on them, and their efforts to maintain functional relationships while working to bring about change. We saw glimpses of their distress on social media and in the tears of Saskatchewan's chief medical health officer at a press conference. The human price of politicizing health was too high, and ultimately the province lost several exceptional clinicians and leaders. The scars left behind will be slow to heal.

Dr. Meili takes us deep into the inner workings of government, the health care system, and his own personal struggle to make a difference in an impossible situation. His deep love for the patients he serves, his colleagues, his province, and its citizens is palpable, and the personal cost of his commitment is generously shared with us.

Trauma evokes many reactions. A common one is to try to forget – to pack away your experience and move forward as though nothing happened. We cannot heal, learn, or change without seeking to understand and process our past. These lessons can show us a path forward and prevent us from repeating past wrongs. Dr. Meili gives us this gift with his book. It is a detailed and passionate reminder of what happened to us – about the struggles and the battles that were fought on behalf of citizens in our hospitals and in the legislature. More importantly, in *A Healthy Future*, Dr. Meili calls on us to do more than remember the past, laying out clear lessons from the COVID-19 pandemic about the path forward to better health for all Canadians. Dr. Courtney Howard has described political involvement as "humanitarian work that is key to a healthy future."[2] By sharing his story of politics as medicine on a larger scale, Dr. Meili shows us why.

A HEALTHY FUTURE

Introduction

> ❝
>
> **It may seem a ridiculous idea, but the only way to fight the plague is with decency.**
>
> – Albert Camus, *The Plague*

The most informative moment of the COVID-19 pandemic in Saskatchewan – the most revealing statement in hundreds of hours of Zoom meetings, press conferences, and livestreams – came down to twenty seconds of silence.

From the beginning of the pandemic and through each subsequent wave, Saskatchewan's chief medical health officer, Dr. Saqib Shahab, was the face and voice of the provincial COVID response. He stands out for how he framed the early days, for occasional statements that clashed with downplaying by his political masters, and for long absences from the public eye that revealed as much about the government's intentions as did the initial daily press conferences. That most striking moment, however, came at the peak of the fourth – or "Delta" – wave, when Saskatchewan's ICUs were overwhelmed to the point that we had to ship patients out of province and ship Armed Forces medical staff in to assist with the local disaster.

During a press conference in which he outlined how intensive care admissions would increase in the weeks ahead, Shahab said, "We've gone so far. We just have to pull along for the next few weeks or months. It is distressing to see what is happening in our ICU and hospitals. And I'm sorry." He stopped for a moment, then choked out, "It's a very challenging time." *Saskatoon StarPhoenix* health reporter Zak Vescera then asked an unusual question: "This wasn't the question I was planning on asking, but Dr. Shahab, are you okay?"

What followed was hard to hear, even though nothing was said. Something about that moment, that particular question, broke through Shahab's renowned composure. For just over twenty seconds, Saskatchewan's chief medical health officer choked back tears and struggled to find his voice. He was not okay, and there was no way to hide it.

Many of us have been there, stoically bearing a burden, able to keep pushing through as long as you're serving the needs of others. Then, when someone does you the kindness of asking you about yourself, the exhaustion hits home and emotions and tears you didn't know were there spring to the surface. In that moment, Dr. Shahab was expressing, against his will, how frustrated and sad he was.

Once he could speak again, Shahab said, "All the evidence is out there. And it's very distressing to see unvaccinated, young, healthy people ending up in ICU and dying ... To see young lives lost through a vaccine-preventable disease – how can we accept this in a country where we've had vaccines available for everyone ever since July?"[1] Along with the reality that people in a wealthy, developed country were refusing a safe, free, effective vaccine, what other frustrations went unspoken, whether it was government interference, health system limitations, or his own fatigue and burnout after a year and a half of spotlights and sleepless nights?

Dr. Shahab's moment of emotional honesty made international headlines. The *Guardian* reported, "Top Saskatchewan health official moved to tears by unchecked COVID spread."[2] Whatever specific blend was troubling him, on that day Shahab channelled what people everywhere were feeling. In his silence, we could hear the exhaustion of health care workers burning out with no help in sight and the grief of people mourning loved ones or afraid for their own health. On some level, his despair gave voice to all those wondering how the worst of our politics had won out when we'd had a chance to make people's well-being a priority again. The experience in Saskatchewan, in our small corner of the country, was a model of the challenges playing out around the world.

A Doctor in Politics

We're all in this together, but we have to stay apart. For many of us, these contrasting notions of solidarity and separation shaped our experience of the pandemic. Crises reveal how strong we can be when challenged and the fragility of so much that we take for granted. *A Healthy Future: Lessons from the Frontlines of a Crisis* explores the story of what happened with COVID-19 in Canada, with a particular focus on Saskatchewan. Our experience of the pandemic can help us understand our strengths and weaknesses and how that knowledge can help us improve the political choices that determine health outcomes.

A deep dive into the stories of one place can tell us about the whole country and the world, just as the story of one patient can tell us about a disease and a health system. This book draws on public events, my personal experiences, and the stories of people whose lives were affected by COVID-19. Some of these stories come from media reports, but most come from interviews with those involved or their family members. The chance to be part of people's lives through medicine, in intimate moments of birth and death, sadness and joy, is an incredible privilege that continually teaches me about what matters most in life. I'm grateful to those who were open with stories that aren't easy to tell and for their permission to share them to shed light on what we can learn from the frontlines of COVID-19.

In February 2021, I was giving vaccines at Merlis Belsher Place, the Saskatoon hockey arena that had been converted into a field hospital (thankfully never used for that purpose) and then a mass immunization centre. A ninety-eight-year-old woman was my first patient of the day. The lower half of our faces were covered by masks, but I could tell, in the way we've all gotten good at telling, that she was beaming. She chatted to me about her childhood, her life on the farm and later in the city, and about the days of the CCF and Tommy Douglas. She had witnessed first-hand the flowering of a political movement coming out of the

Second World War, where ordinary citizens demanded their share of the nation's wealth in the form of social programs. Universal health insurance, or Medicare, was the crown jewel. She apologized for talking so much (unnecessarily, of course; I was charmed) and said it was her first real outing in almost a year. Her eyes lit up as she talked about seeing grandkids and neighbours again.

Later that same month, while on the COVID-19 internal medicine service at Royal University Hospital (RUH), I was called to the observation ward to pronounce the death of an eighty-eight-year-old man from Saskatoon. Before coming to the hospital, he had been living independently, still driving, still making all his own meals. He had been very careful during the pandemic, doing his best to stay safe. His bad luck was catching the virus from someone who came to help him with a few chores at home. I looked into his eyes, checked for his pulse, and confirmed that he was indeed gone. I then sat down to fill out the appropriate paperwork. At the front of his chart was the phone number of his daughter in Alberta. It was five in the morning, but the note said to call any time. She knew immediately who was calling and why. Through her tears she described the heartbreak of losing her father without having been able to visit, without being able to say goodbye.

Family doctor and political leader is an unusual combination, and one that has coloured my experience of the pandemic. After being elected as a Member of the Legislative Assembly (MLA) in Saskatoon Meewasin in 2017, I kept doing occasional clinical shifts, filling in at my former practice at the West Side Community Clinic or helping out at REACH, the refugee clinic run by my wife, Mahli Brindamour, and her colleagues in pediatrics and family medicine. When I became leader of the New Democratic Party (NDP) of Saskatchewan in 2018, I switched to an inactive medical licence and stopped doing any clinical service. Then along came COVID-19, and it was clear that we would need all hands on deck and that anyone who could help out should step up. I called the College of Physicians and Surgeons of Saskatchewan and started the process to sharpen my skills and pitch in where I could.

The path to family medicine and social democracy wasn't obvious growing up. My two older brothers, Miles and Jim, and I were raised on a farm near Courval, Saskatchewan – population never more than twenty in my lifetime and single digits for a long time now. For those with a sense of Saskatchewan geography, if you draw a line from Mossbank to Mortlach, our farm is where that line crosses Highway 363 between Moose Jaw and Gravelbourg. It was a mixed cattle and grain farm while we were growing up, then switched over to just grain (durum, lentils, chickpeas, canola, etc.). My father operated it for over thirty years. Jim is the farmer now. As kids, we took the bus to school in Coderre, twelve miles to the east. Later we moved to Moose Jaw, where I attended St. Agnes School and Vanier Collegiate for the end of elementary and high school.

After an unfocused first attempt at the University of Saskatchewan – and the grades to match – I took some time off to work and to think. I decided that life is short, eternity long, and that I wanted to do something good with my time in the world. I wanted to serve, to help the people most in need, and I became interested in health and in social justice. I'm aware that's a term that's been much maligned, but in my world view, faith, and profession of medicine, there is no higher calling than to work to make the world more fair and to have a "preferential option" for the poorest and most vulnerable among us. I thought briefly about politics at the time, attracted to the chance to influence policy for the greater good, but decided I was too impatient. I thought medicine would mean a more immediate impact, that I could see the change in people's lives in real time rather than wait decades. I had the idea that the job of a doctor is making friends all day. You sit down with people, hear their stories, help in whatever way you can, and go away having made a meaningful connection.

With that new goal in mind, I started over at university, much more motivated to study hard. After a couple of tries, I convinced the College of Medicine to give me a shot. In medical school, we learned the clinical and communication skills we would need to serve our patients well. We also learned about the social determinants of health, the upstream factors – political factors – that have the biggest impact on health. As Director-General of the World Health Organization Tedros Adhanom Ghebreyesus recently wrote, "Health does not begin in clinics or hospitals any more than justice begins in law courts or peace starts on the battlefield. Rather, health starts with the conditions in which we are born and raised, and in schools, streets, workplaces, homes, markets, water sources, kitchens, and in the very air we breathe."[3] More than any lecture or article, it was time spent volunteering or studying in Brazil, Nicaragua, India, Zambia, and Mozambique, as well as Northern Saskatchewan and inner-city Saskatoon, that brought those lessons home. You can't see real poverty, see the gross unfairness of a world where so many are born without any chance of a healthy life, and look at health as just a matter of doctors and nurses, hospitals and pharmacies ever again.

After completing my training in Saskatoon, I practised as a family doctor for a decade. First, I worked as a locum physician, filling in for a week or two in small towns like Kelvington, Arcola, Leader, and Maidstone, with the intimidatingly full-scope practice that is rural medicine. I worked for the College of Medicine setting up the Making the Links program, giving students an opportunity to learn in Northern Saskatchewan (Île-à-la-Crosse, Buffalo River Dene Nation, Pinehouse), at the SWITCH clinic in inner-city Saskatoon, and in rural Mozambique. For several years before getting elected, I worked as part of the team at the West Side Community Clinic on 20th Street in Saskatoon, with a focus on obstetrics, HIV, and addictions medicine.

And that naive notion of making friends all day? Well, it was exactly right. I loved getting to know my patients, counselling them through a tough time, meeting their new baby with them, even saying goodbye with their families when it was the end. There were so many beautiful, sad, joyful, and funny moments. At the same time, the frustration was constant, especially when working with underserved communities. As much as I could help out with a prescription or a referral, with good advice or just a listening ear, patients go back to the conditions that make them sick in the first place. Unless we're addressing the root causes of illness, we see a revolving door for the health system and constant and chronic illness for people and their communities.

The legendary German pathologist and statesman Rudolf Virchow once said that "Medicine is a social science, and politics is nothing more than medicine on a large scale."[4] I took that concept to heart, first running for leader of the Saskatchewan NDP in 2009 and again in 2013, finishing a close second in both races. Between those contests, I wrote a book called *A Healthy Society: How a Focus on Health Can Revive Canadian Democracy.*[5] I then worked with a team to start Upstream,[6] an organization dedicated to promoting the concept of the social determinants of health as a guide to improving our political choices, and helped establish the Division of Social Accountability at the University of Saskatchewan's College of Medicine.[7] In 2017, I ran for an NDP nomination and then in a provincial by-election to become the MLA for Saskatoon Meewasin. Once elected, I was surprised and pleased to discover how much the two roles had in common: meeting people, helping in small ways, advocating for change. Making friends every day carried over into public life. Of course, in politics you make enemies as well, exposing yourself to much more scrutiny and controversy, taking positions and making decisions that cannot please everyone.

While the line between politics and medicine is porous, the irony is not lost on me that *A Healthy Society* came out as I was leaving medicine for electoral politics and this one follows on my leaving political office to return to medicine. I was elected leader of the Saskatchewan NDP in March 2018. Two years later, after scrambling as best I could up the steep learning curve of the job, I found myself in what we all found ourselves in: a global pandemic. COVID-19 disrupted our lives in ways we couldn't predict and still don't fully comprehend.

A family doctor leading the opposition in what would turn out to be arguably the least scientifically informed pandemic response in the country was a role that was at once uniquely challenging and so appropriate as to be a bit too on the nose. While continuing my work in politics, I returned to medical practice, helping out with vaccine delivery, COVID assessment, hospital care, and clinics in the community. Through multiple waves and the political demands of legislative sessions, a provincial election, and the daily news cycle, I did my best to maintain the focus on the health of the people I was there to serve. In *A Healthy Future,* I speak from that vantage point of family doc turned politician turned strange mixture of both, telling the story of COVID-19 in Saskatchewan and Canada and exploring how what we learned from the experience should inform our next steps.

Moving Upstream

In *A Healthy Society*, I argued that health should be our primary goal. The best measure of success of any government is the quality and distribution of good health among the people they have been elected to serve. If that's the goal, then we have to ask, What policy choices will help us achieve it?

There's a classic public health parable that imagines child after child floating helplessly in a river and people realizing that they need to do more than fish them out. They need to head upstream and find out who keeps chucking the kids in the water in the first place. The story of the babies in the river is not a new one; it's a stitch in time, an ounce of prevention, a fence at the top of the cliff rather than an ambulance at the bottom. Folk wisdom and empirical evidence agree: keeping people healthy is much less expensive and much more effective than treating the sick. When we address the root causes of illness, we relieve the stress and pressure on the systems of reaction, the emergency rooms and surgical suites, the shelters and food banks, and we move our city, province, or nation further away from illness and despair.

The social determinants of health, using the Canadian list compiled by York University professor Dr. Dennis Raphael, are income and income distribution, education, unemployment and job security, employment and working conditions, early childhood development, food insecurity, housing, social exclusion, social safety net, health services, geography, disability, Indigenous ancestry, gender, immigration, race, and globalization.[8] These are the upstream factors with the biggest impact on whether people will be sick or well, whether their lives will be short or long. Former Saskatchewan premier Roy Romanow spoke of this concept as the third revolution in public health: "Historians tell us that we have had two great revolutions in the course of public health. The first was the control of infectious diseases, notwithstanding some recent challenges. The second was the battle against non-communicable diseases. I believe that the third revolution is about moving from an illness model to focusing on all the things that promote well-being."[9]

When we undertake interventions that decrease income inequality, we also decrease heart disease and stroke. When we tackle food security, we tackle diabetes. When we improve literacy, we improve life expectancy. We save lives, and we save money. Investments today pay off over time in lowered health, social services, and justice costs, in economic productivity. This is not a new idea; the body of evidence for it is overwhelming. The problem is those two words, *over time.* The savings may be enormous, the quality of life for the beneficiaries incredible, but those investments, just like putting money in your savings account or RRSPs, come at the expense of today's spending priorities. How do we convince people, particularly those who feel their elected positions depend on today's purchases, not tomorrow's savings, that the payoff is real and worth the wait?

Usually, when we talk about that investment in literacy paying off in life expectancy, that's a ten-, twenty-, or forty-year payoff. The return on investment is enormous, but the realization is long. And then along came COVID-19, and the risk-and-reward, call-and-response curve went from decades to weeks or even days. Choices about public health measures like masks and vaccines could mean the difference between life and death, between inconvenience and disruption and a completely over- whelmed health care system. A mask mandate on Monday decreased transmissions in a week, hospitalizations in two, and deaths in four. A new variant ignored in June overwhelmed hospitals in September. The river was flowing so fast.

We learned so much, so quickly, and then seemed to unlearn it even faster.

Like no other time in our collective memory, COVID-19 has laid bare just how much health matters. When our health is threatened, everything else grinds to a halt. We know this in our own lives, whether it's staying home when sick or shifting our priorities completely when a loved one is seriously ill. In 2020 we saw this on a grand scale as the entire world went on sick leave. And just as how well you can take care of yourself and your family is determined by what kind of supports you have at work and at home, how well countries were able to care for their people said a lot about their resources and priorities. Returning to Raphael's list, it's clear that COVID followed that same distribution, affecting those living in poverty or without social support much more, and leaving those with stable housing and a good education less at risk. New diseases are very good at finding pre-existing fault lines and exploiting them.

The Trouble with Normal

By the end of 2022, nearly 50,000 people had died from COVID across Canada, with nearly 2,000 of those in Saskatchewan. The latter number may not seem so high, but in a province of 1.2 million, it puts us at the third-highest death rate in the country, well above the national average. It also means nearly everyone in the province knows someone who died or was hospitalized with a serious illness, or lost someone they loved to COVID. And it may be far more. Dr. Tara Moriarty of the University of Toronto has been calculating excess deaths throughout the pandemic and estimates that thousands of COVID-19 deaths have gone undetected or unreported.[10]

It may be years before we have the final tally of official and estimated deaths, but one thing is clear. Whatever the number, it's too high. Canada was hit far worse than necessary and Saskatchewan was far from unscathed, with among the worst second, third, and fourth waves in the country.

Variants and vaccines changed the game. People have lost the masks, ditched the distance, and moved on. You'll notice I don't say "gone back to normal," because so much of normal wasn't great, and that's been revealed by the havoc the pandemic played with our lives. COVID didn't cause the problems in our emergency rooms, our ICUs, our long-term care homes, our homeless shelters, our schools, our town squares. It revealed those problems, exacerbated them, made them – at least for a time – impossible to ignore. "At least for a time" is the operative phrase here. "Brain fog" is one of the symptoms described post-COVID, but there is also a time fog that has affected us all. Things are moving so quickly that we have a hard time remembering the present, let alone the past few chaotic years.

We need to peer back through that fog to understand what happened if we are to learn and apply the lessons of this age-defining period. The collision of a worldwide infectious outbreak, ecological devastation and the resulting natural disasters, and a destabilizing war in Europe has led some to describe the current moment as an era of polycrisis. Stories from the frontlines of the COVID crisis – from those whose lives were on the line to those charged with leading us through troubled times – help us

Introduction

learn lessons we can't live without as we face an increasingly uncertain future.

COVID-19 has been devastating, disruptive, tragic, and confusing. There's nothing we can do to undo the trauma of this disease or bring back the lives claimed. We can honour them by insisting we take the time to learn from the loss. Our great task now is to refuse the temptation to turn it all off and move on as quickly as we can, and to instead dig into what went wrong, what went right, and how we can use what this moment taught us to do better. Our task is, as always, to build a healthy future.

First Wave

MARCH–AUGUST 2020

What's true of all the evils in the world
is true of plague as well.
It helps men to rise above themselves.

– Albert Camus, *The Plague*

Total cases in Canada	129,594
Total cases in Saskatchewan	1,622
Deaths from COVID in Canada	9,139
Deaths from COVID in Saskatchewan	24

Provincial Public Health Measures

March 13, 2020   Public gatherings restricted to 250 people

March 16, 2020   Hospital and long-term care visitors limited to essential visitors only

International travellers required to self-isolate and self-monitor for fourteen days upon return to the province

March 18, 2020   Provincial state of emergency declared

March 20, 2020   K–12 classes suspended

Public gatherings restricted to twenty-five people

Mandatory fourteen-day self-isolation for positive cases and close contacts

March 25, 2020   Public gatherings limited to ten people

Non-essential businesses and public facilities closed

March 26, 2020   Private gatherings restricted to ten people

May 7, 2020   School year cancelled

Gathering Clouds

November 17, 2019	First known case of COVID-19 is detected in a fifty-five-year-old man from Wuhan, China
December 7, 2019	Wuhan doctors record first suspected case of human-to-human transmission of COVID-19
January 13, 2020	First case of COVID-19 outside China is found; a woman in Thailand is quarantined
January 15, 2020	The World Health Organization (WHO) describes coronavirus as transmissible from person to person[1]
January 21, 2020	First case of COVID-19 in the United States is found in Washington state
January 25, 2020	Canada reports first case of COVID-19 linked to travel in Wuhan

From time to time, we hear of local outbreaks of known deadly illnesses like cholera or Ebola, or the emergence of new viral illnesses popping up in other parts of the world. Often, in the midst of our busy lives, we pay no attention at all. Perhaps in a better moment we get curious, read a little bit more, maybe donate some money to a relief organization or to medical research. We might even have a flash of guilty gratitude that it's not happening here. But for the most part, an outbreak or epidemic halfway around the world is someone else's problem, and we have problems of our own that are taking up our time. It's human nature to attend to what's close at hand and tangible, not to some far-off country to which we have no personal connection. Today has enough trouble in it, and our immediate surroundings do as well.

In the spring of 2020, a whisper from across the world, the leap of a single subcellular organism from another species to ours, disrupted human life in every corner of the planet. The first days of the coronavirus crisis set the pattern for how Canada would respond and how badly our communities would be impacted. As a doctor in the house, practising politics through a health lens, I found myself in a unique position. My view, heavy as it is on the events in the Saskatchewan legislature, may seem narrow, but it reveals how things started and the patterns being formed that would play themselves out over the entire pandemic.

The whisper started a long way away, and at first seemed to have little to do with our lives here in Canada. The first known case of an atypical viral pneumonia, later attributed to a novel coronavirus that would come to be known as SARS-CoV-2, was detected in a fifty-five-year-old man from Wuhan, China, in November 2019. On December 7 of the same year, doctors in Wuhan recorded the first suspected case of human-to-human transmission of the virus. My local newspaper, the *Saskatoon StarPhoenix*, had its first story on coronavirus on January 10, reporting that "a mystery virus has been identified as the cause of a cluster of nearly 60 pneumonia cases in China that have put health authorities around the world on high alert."[2]

A woman in Thailand was quarantined with coronavirus on January 13, the first case outside China. On the 21st, the first case was confirmed in North America, in Washington state. And less than a week later saw Canada's first case: a traveller from Wuhan tested positive in British Columbia. No one could say whether we were dealing with something that would spread quickly around the world, like H1N1 in 2010, or that would be deadlier but more easily contained, like the earlier coronavirus outbreaks of SARS in 2003, or something else entirely. What was clear was that the situation was changing rapidly and, rather than an isolated local concern, was destined to be a global disruption.

The lightning-fast transmission of a new disease to an unprepared world was, of course, the most striking evidence of that interconnection. But we also saw worldwide shifts in consumer demand and disrupted supply chains. We all remember shelves empty of toilet paper as panic buying in parts of Asia spread around the world. We saw food supply chains disrupted, as restaurant closures changed markets overnight and outbreaks in meat-packing plants in nearby states and provinces left shelves empty. This threatened supply in places like Saskatchewan that – despite producing enormous amounts of food – have lost much of the capacity to process it to the point of consumption. And, in later months, new variants of the virus would emerge in countries that had been over-whelmed by COVID-19, endangering the recovery of places that had initially been more successful in their control of the virus. This further demonstrated that in a global pandemic, our local efforts matter, but so do the efforts (and support for them) in every part of the world.

I won't pretend to have had any understanding of what that first word of a new illness in China would mean for Saskatchewan, Canada, or the world. No one did. But on January 25, the first case of what was then known as the novel coronavirus was confirmed in Canada, and I was concerned enough to phone the office of then Saskatchewan min-ister of health Jim Reiter and ask about our province's plan. He invited me and NDP health critic Vicki Mowat to meet with him and Dr. Saqib Shahab, Saskatchewan's chief medical health officer (CMHO).

I didn't know Dr. Shahab well at the time, though our paths had crossed once or twice. We first met as part of a provincial discussion on how to address the province's HIV crisis. (Saskatchewan still leads the country in new HIV cases per capita, three times the national average and nearly double the rate of the next highest province.[3]) I also knew of him through his son, Izn Shahab, who is completing his residency in neurology. As a medical student, Izn worked with me on a study that explored the social factors behind "no-shows" – the patients that book appointments but for some reason don't make it to the clinic.[4] Little did I know how much we'd all get to know Dr. Shahab, and CMHOs across Canada, and what prominent and important roles they would play in all of our lives in the weeks and months ahead.

In that first briefing, Minister Reiter assured us that work was underway on a plan to respond to the pandemic that built on the 2009–10 H1N1 pandemic response. He also offered regular updates and collaborative work in response to the coronavirus. I left the meeting with some hope that, at least on this one issue, we could be guided by evidence, set partisanship aside, and work together on behalf of the health of the people we were elected to serve.

The minister's avowed commitment to get ahead of the coronavirus did not translate into action. Later we would learn that not a single extra dollar was spent in public health[5] – a sector that had seen repeated cuts over the preceding decade – prior to the declaration of a state of emergency on March 18. We also learned that essential equipment like ventilators and hospital beds had not been ordered until mid-March,[6] and in some cases not until after a state of emergency had been declared. Epidemiologist Dr. Nazeem Muhajarine was critical of those choices, saying, "We are flatlanders. We can see storms brewing miles ahead. And we knew this storm was brewing since early January. If you're a good farmer and you can see the storm coming you protect your flock, you take what steps are needed to protect your crop, your flock, everything."[7]

The biggest barrier to preparation and collaboration was that, while the rest of the world was planning for a pandemic, Premier Scott Moe and the Saskatchewan Party were planning a snap election. The Sask Party had started as a coalition of right-of-centre Liberals and Progressive Conservatives who had to change their name after nearly bankrupting Saskatchewan under Grant Devine. Back in 2007, the day after Brad Wall was elected premier, he announced his plan to fulfill his election promise of set election dates. It's something he still refers to as evidence of how governments should behave, citing it as recently as fall 2020 as evidence that "they did what they said they would do."[8] It was a valuable change, one that could level the playing field and, as Sask Party cabinet minister Don Morgan said, "remove some of the political gamesmanship and voter cynicism we have seen in the past."[9]

Just over a year earlier, Scott Moe had stated his commitment to following the set election date legislation and his appreciation for the fairness it represented. But that commitment was out the window as Sask Party strategists thought they had a chance to surprise the opposition, and it was full steam ahead for a spring election. The plan was to deliver a budget in mid-March to kick off an April election, and it was the worst-kept secret in the province. Candidates were nominated, ads were running, Elections Saskatchewan was booking space for polling stations (we would later learn they found themselves competing with the Saskatchewan Health Authority (SHA), who were trying to book the same spaces for COVID testing),[10] and we were all preparing for the door knocking, handshaking, rallies, and debates to follow. Needless to say, there was a surprise in store for us all, but it was a lot more impactful than a snap election.

A Global Emergency

January 31, 2020	WHO declares the novel coronavirus a global emergency
February 6, 2020	Canadians are evacuated from Wuhan
February 7, 2020	Dr. Li Wenliang, early COVID-19 whistleblower, dies from the virus in Wuhan
February 10, 2020	Worldwide COVID-19 death toll surpasses SARS at 900; the virus is present in twenty-seven countries
February 11, 2020	WHO names coronavirus SARS-CoV-2 and the illness it causes COVID-19
February 26, 2020	Virus spreads quickly around the world; Iran and Italy are hit hard
February 28, 2020	Scott Moe cites coronavirus as reason for possible early election call
March 9, 2020	First Canadian dies after contracting COVID-19 at Lynn Valley Care Centre in North Vancouver
	Italy enters nationwide lockdown
March 11, 2020	Federal health minister Patty Hajdu calls COVID-19 a "national emergency and crisis," and urges people to stay home[11]
	WHO declares COVID-19 a pandemic

March 12, 2020	US president Donald Trump suspends air travel from Europe
	NBA and NHL suspend seasons
	Asymptomatic transmission of SARS-CoV-2 is reported
	Ontario closes schools
	Sophie Grégoire Trudeau, Tom Hanks test positive for COVID-19
	Ottawa unveils $1 billion in pandemic funding
	First presumptive COVID-19 case is found in Saskatchewan

On March 12, I was invited to address the delegates at the annual convention of the Saskatchewan Association of Rural Municipalities (SARM). It's no secret that the political fortunes of New Democrats in rural Saskatchewan have been disappointing in recent years, meaning this could be a tough crowd. In fact, it had been many years since a leader of the Opposition had been invited to speak, and on an ordinary day, I might have been nervous about the reception.

On an ordinary day, I would have started off talking about my own rural roots, about growing up on the family farm in the Rural Municipality of Rodgers, near Courval, where my brother Jim still farms today. I might have spoken about working as a family doctor all over rural Saskatchewan and the frustration of how decisions made in the legislature, not in the emergency room, make the biggest difference in people's health. I'd have talked about how we need to work to address upstream factors if we want to keep people healthy. I would have then described how our plans would improve life in rural Saskatchewan compared with those of our opponents. You know, a standard political speech. Ordinary.

But this was no ordinary day. It was something completely new. This was March 12, 2020, the day it hit home that all of our lives had changed. We didn't yet know how much, or for how long. We still don't, I suppose. But that day in March we knew it had hit for real.

The day before, the World Health Organization had declared COVID-19 a pandemic. A pandemic is "an epidemic occurring world-wide, or over a very wide area, crossing international boundaries and usually affecting a large number of people."[12] That classification made it clear: the new coronavirus would not be confined to one part of the world. It would spread everywhere.

The first confirmed case of COVID-19 in Saskatchewan was announced that day, found in a resident in their sixties who had just returned from Egypt. The first Canadian had died from the virus a few days earlier. Then US president Donald Trump, after initially dismissing the virus, had banned air travel from Europe. The upcoming Juno awards in Saskatoon were cancelled. The NBA season was suspended. Tim Hortons had cancelled Roll Up the Rim. It was a very big deal.

I told the audience that it was not a time to panic, not a time to buy a lifetime's supply of toilet paper, but that it was time to act. And I described an idea, novel on that day, that we'd all get used to hearing: it was time to flatten the curve.

There are two possible distribution curves for infections in an out-break: either one that spikes, meaning the virus is reaching those it will infect quickly, or one that is long and flat, meaning it's moving more slowly through the population. With all the cases at once, the high spike curve, you get higher mortality, more health care workers are sick, health care services are overwhelmed – it's a disaster.

When the cases are spread out over time – the flat curve – more health care resources are available, there are potentially fewer cases overall, and there is lower mortality for those who do get sick. We may even be lucky enough to get into the vaccination and dedicated treatment window, as scientists everywhere, including at the VIDO-InterVac vaccine lab at the University of Saskatchewan in Saskatoon, were already hard at work seeking cures and vaccines.[13]

Key to that goal was another concept that was brand new to our vocabulary then but now seems so obvious: social distancing. We would later talk more of physical distancing, as we tried to emphasize avoiding the contact that could lead to infection but still reaching out in other ways to avoid loneliness and separation. When it came to distancing, Saskatchewan had some natural advantages. My favourite COVID T-shirt was one that read "Saskatchewan, physical distancing since 1905." On my family's farm, the next neighbour is a couple of miles away. Even in our largest cities, we don't have the density of the world's metropolises. While the number of people living in unstable housing has risen in recent years, most people in the province live in safe, clean housing. These factors protect us, but only if we're careful, only if we do everything we can to reduce community transmission and make the extra efforts to keep the virus out of congregate living settings like homeless shelters, long-term care homes, and prisons.

In my speech to SARM, I called on the government to invite municipal leaders like the delegates present and their urban counterparts, First Nations and Métis leaders, leaders in K–12 and post-secondary education, in health, labour, and business to form an all-party, all-hands-on-deck table to start our response to COVID off right. Of all the calls to government that went ignored and unanswered during that period, this was the biggest missed opportunity. It was the moment we went into silos and guaranteed the political polarization of the pandemic response.

Thinking back to that day in front of SARM, with a crowd of hundreds of people from every corner of our province, it's wild to imagine how we went overnight from gatherings of that size to many months apart. Despite the challenging message, people were ready to hear it. At that moment, while we were sending everyone to their separate corners, there was a heightened sense that we were all in this together. That we were about to face something massive and that it was going to take all of us. That in the face of such a challenge, there was a chance to look beyond whatever we thought divided us toward a common goal of getting through this with as many of us alive and well as possible. This has been challenged since, as missed opportunities and misinformation have reinforced and even worsened pre-existing polarization. Still, thinking back to that moment, to that supposedly tough crowd listening intently and ready to do what was necessary to keep themselves and their neighbours safe, reminds me that there is common ground and common purpose in most of us if we are willing to seek it out.

Our Separate Ways

The separation of the months to follow made that harder, as we didn't find ourselves in rooms full of new faces. We didn't shake hands with strangers. We didn't get to do the classic Saskatchewan social dance of finding out whom you know in common, how few degrees of separation there are between each of us. We now have work to do to make those connections again, and hopefully an even greater appetite to make them.

On that day, however, I urged everyone to skip the handshake. I joked that as a politician that was an extra burden: working the room is half the job description. It was indeed strange to, for the first time, refuse an outstretched hand. We all want to show each other respect and attention with a friendly, hearty handshake. But as one of the reeves reached out by reflex, I slid my hand in my pocket, said an awkward thanks for having me, and headed back to the legislature.

Just the day before, on March 11, I'd seen Jeremy Harrison, the minister of the economy and one of the main decision-makers in the government benches, walking out to the MLA parking spaces in front of the Legislative Building. I caught up with him as he was climbing into his truck and urged him, for reasons of public safety, to reconsider the snap election. He brushed it off, saying something like it's always the same – Zika, West Nile Virus, there's always something that's going to kill us all and nothing ever happens.

Our opposition team had asked about this several times in the Legislative Assembly and, while Premier Moe had changed from his original position that the coronavirus epidemic was a good reason to call a snap election, he was digging in his heels on his plan to go to the polls that spring.[14] The members on his side hadn't just resisted being responsible and calling it off: they'd laughed out loud at the idea, heckling the very notion that we should be concerned. The minister for rural and remote health yelled, "What if, what if," from his seat, as though the notion of acting to prevent a disaster was ridiculous. The minister of finance referred to me and my Opposition colleagues as "Doctor Doom and his whole caucus of gloom."[15] One gets used to this behaviour from the government members – the legislature is not a civil place and having a large majority brings out their schoolyard bully tendencies – but it was shocking to hear at such a serious moment.

The idea that, in the context of an emerging, dangerous infectious disease, we would send people door to door shaking hands, holding rallies, and then all gathering in polling stations on election day was inconceivable. If you were looking for a way to make sure the virus spread as quickly as possible, that's what you'd do. It's the opposite of physical distancing and would have been tremendously dangerous, not only for Saskatchewan but for the containment efforts of the entire country. Public health physician Dr. Anne Huang boldly wrote a public letter calling on the government to stop this foolish plan, describing elections as "exercises in reducing social distances" and making it clear that "containing COVID-19 requires a massive societal response, strong government leadership and social-distancing measures. Calling a snap election this spring has the potential to expose a lot of people to the virus and will make a coordinated response in Saskatchewan more difficult."[16]

Of course, the election wasn't our team's only, or even our main, concern. Above all, we wanted to see a plan to keep people safe and to make sure our health care system was able to handle the strain of an onslaught of new admissions. When Vicki Mowat asked about a plan, it turned out the minister of health had not followed up on his commitments from our earlier meeting: there wasn't one. Despite his repeated claims in the house that there was, our office learned through a freedom of information request that it wasn't the case. Instead, a mad scramble at the ministry that night had produced a few slides of a PowerPoint presentation showing a warmed-over version of the H1N1 strategy being presented as a master plan the following day.[17] This is the pattern that would continue throughout the pandemic, a government that would overestimate its preparedness while downplaying the seriousness of the threat.

Along with a plan for prevention and a response to health system challenges, we called for a budget that reflected the new world we were in. But there too we saw a government reluctant to let go of the world they thought they were living in, a world where they were presenting a balanced budget and had everything handily in control. The problem was that the budget had been finalized weeks before and reflected neither the worldwide economic crash nor the need for massive expenditures to support Saskatchewan people.

Now there's no question this was a very difficult time to be preparing a budget. It was a difficult time to be planning for a new, dangerous viral illness. Mistakes will be made. That's normal. The challenge for governments of all stripes is to find out how we can move beyond "everything I do is good; I can show no weakness" to "we are giving this everything we have and would like your help to do it better." A tremendous amount of goodwill and a real opportunity to do better was wasted in the hyperpartisanship of our current polarized public discourse, and the planned snap election set us off on the wrong foot from day one.

It didn't have to be that way, and there were already Canadian examples of a better approach.[18] Dwight Ball, premier of Newfoundland and Labrador, established an all-party committee that included the leaders of the provincial opposition parties. Opposition leaders were included in Prince Edward Island's "COVID-19 response table." And on March 12, the day after the first case of COVID-19 was discovered in the province, New Brunswick premier Blaine Higgs swore the leaders of the three opposition parties – one of whom didn't even have a seat in the legislature – into his cabinet as part of a committee that included the ministers of public safety, social development, education, and health. That spring and summer, the different party leaders met and, under the confidentiality of cabinet, decided together on the best course of action. Notably, New Brunswick had one of the country's best responses to COVID-19 as part of the Atlantic Bubble.

Regina Leader-Post columnist Murray Mandryk suggested a similar approach here in Saskatchewan. "The buy-in to the tough-but-justifiable measures imposed by the Saskatchewan Party government needs to be accompanied by an entirely different all-party approach to governance that brings in not only NDP Opposition Leader Ryan Meili but also major civic leaders like Regina Mayor Michael Fougere and Saskatoon Mayor Charlie Clark."[19] University of Regina professor Howard Leeson went further, evoking the First World War unity cabinet and writing that "Premier Moe should immediately constitute a special cabinet committee that deals with the coronavirus in its entirety. This committee should operate unlike other cabinet committees. It should be staffed only in part by traditional civil servants but should bring in a wide variety of advisers from the whole community. It should include the leader of the Opposition, Ryan Meili, since he is a medical doctor."[20]

Our initial meeting with Dr. Shahab and the health minister had given me some hope that we might see some such cross-partisan collective action. I don't know if this collaboration didn't happen as a hangover from the snap election planning, a shift in focus to the now coming fall election, or simply a super-majority government whose ministers frequently say in question period that they will "take no lessons from the members opposite." While there would have been a need for criticism and difference along the way, some of the polarization and animosity – not just between ruling and opposition parties but between Saskatchewan people – could have been eased with a signal of unity. That inability to put partisanship aside gave the people of Saskatchewan an unbalanced COVID response and contributed to the poor outcomes and heightened social tension that would follow.

Heading Home

March 13, 2020	Canadians are advised against all non-essential international travel
	Toronto Stock Exchange sees largest single-day drop since 1940
March 16, 2020	Dow Jones sees largest drop in history
	Major national travel restrictions go into effect
	Saskatchewan schools to close March 20
March 17, 2020	Alberta and Ontario declare states of emergency
	Trump tells Americans to avoid gatherings, eating in restaurants; oil prices plummet; deaths in Italy continue to rise; France goes into lockdown
March 18, 2020	State of emergency declared in Saskatchewan
	Gatherings of more than fifty people are banned
	Fitness centres, casinos, and bingo halls are ordered closed

March 18 was our last day in the legislature that spring. States of emergency had been declared in Alberta and Ontario. Saskatchewan and the rest of the country soon followed suit. This included a ban on gatherings over fifty, which meant it only made sense to end the session. This is something on which both sides of the house could agree. There would be time to figure out how to resume the work of the legislature, but now it was time to go home, be safe, and set an example. Question period the day before had been a sombre affair, ending with promises to work together.

The spirit of collaboration never took root, with things taking a strange turn in Regina that day. Despite being clear that a budget written in January made no sense in March, the government insisted on plowing ahead, at least partially. Their plan was to instead release a half budget, one that described expenditures but didn't include revenues, then adjourn the assembly. I don't know of any example of something like that being done before, here or anywhere. A budget that announces what will be spent without saying what was being gained or borrowed is simply out of step with the principles of fiscal management and the rules of the legislature.

Early that morning, Jeremy Harrison (the same government house leader who thought we were overreacting to COVID-19 and compared it to Zika and West Nile) called Cathy Sproule, the opposition house leader, and told her there was suspected community transmission of COVID-19 and the government would declare a state of emergency. I'll never forget the sense of betrayal we felt that day. Here was a government that recognized things were bad enough to declare a state of emergency, something none of us had ever seen in our lives, but wanted to put off the announcement until after their feel-good half-budget press conference and farewell speeches in the house. I texted the premier the following, hoping he would change course:

> We understand that the government has had information of increased case numbers and community transmission since last night. If this is the case, it's irresponsible to keep this information from the public. People are at work and in situations of public exposure. I expect this information to be released immediately. The Minister and the CMHO and you, as premier, have a duty to inform the public now.

He didn't respond and they went ahead with their media event as though nothing had changed.

Once the word was out, plans for big speeches in the assembly were shelved. We gathered for all of four minutes, just long enough to agree to adjourn. The heat and bluster of parliamentary debate gave way to a strange and quiet retreat to our own corners. An awkward stream of MLAs and staff headed out to their cars, the same sort of scene that was playing out at workplaces and schools around the world. Usually, at the end of session, the two sides meet on the assembly floor and shake hands, like a line of hockey players saying, "Good game." There are always a few so fiercely partisan that they can't bring themselves to fraternize even that lightly with the enemy, but most of us take that moment to recognize we are all doing hard jobs and wish each other well despite our differences. That day, for obvious reasons, we parted with no hugs or handshakes. The premier and I quickly did our post-session scrums with reporters. I urged people to remember that whatever our political leanings, we had a common enemy in the virus.[21] Each member then quickly gathered their things and quietly headed down the marble steps of the legislature to find their families and figure out how to deal with a new, unknown world.

The Longest March

COVID-19 has done funny things to our perception of time. People talk without irony about the "before-times," and waves six months earlier seem like ancient history compared to whatever news is bearing down upon us now.

There is likely no other period that stands out in our memories – and in that warped perception of time – in quite the same way as March and April 2020. The word "quarantine" comes from "forty" in Italian – *quarantina*, which referred to the forty days of isolation required for ships landing during the Black Death and symbolized the forty days of self-denial and sacrifice of Lent. Schools were closed and the streets were nearly empty. The stores that were still open had hardly a soul in them. People truly were staying home. At once brief and exhaustingly long, those forty days in the spring of 2020 stand out as the most intense and life-changing period of the pandemic, the period when we stayed apart and felt together.

The world stood still in a way none of us had ever experienced. Restaurants, gyms, and all kinds of stores closed their doors. So did schools and, to a large degree, clinics and hospitals. Drop-off care packages, drive-by visits, and shouted window exchanges were the extent of our in-person social engagements. Collective action and curtailment of personal liberties for the greater good were quickly accepted, more out of concern for others than for fear for oneself. And the level of uncertainty had almost everyone, even many who would go on to become staunch opponents of public health measures, fully engaged in the project of flattening the curve, of staying home and staying safe.

There was an incredible sense of being all together in a remarkable moment. It was scary, but in some ways exhilarating. I'm reluctant to go too easily to war analogies – no one was bombing our homes – but there was something of the camaraderie of times of conflict, the community spirit of a London under blitz. Ironically, the tensions between people would become much greater after that period of isolation. We were more together when we were apart, more polarized as we came back together. That March, however, there was something of that "keep calm and carry on" spirit in the air along with the novel virus.

COVID Kindness

That spirit manifested as kindness, ranging from neighbourly acts like dropping off groceries or calling to check in on a lonely senior, to larger volunteer efforts. Saskatchewan people have a reputation for charitable acts, with the highest percentage in the country of people who do volunteer work.[1] The annual telethon TeleMiracle, with its catchphrases of "Ring those phones" and "Where are we going? Higher!," is an incredibly successful fundraiser for the Kinsmen Foundation and a cultural touchstone for the province's charitable sensibilities. This community spirit was on full display in the early days of the pandemic. Dr. Theresa Tam, Canada's chief public health officer, tweeted out thanks to the Reverse School Bus project in Regina.[2] This was an initiative of Regina teacher Kam Bahia, who teamed up with her brother's restaurant, the Lobby Kitchen and Bar, to deliver meals to students who would normally be accessing school lunch programs.

In Prince Albert, seventy-nine-year-old Eleanor Land baked dozens of loaves of bread a week for the Community Cares Kitchen, a new not-for-profit founded to provide meals to vulnerable people. When Eleanor's oven broke from overuse, the organizers of the kitchen were only too happy to raise the money to get her back baking.[3]

Angela Bishop, a Métis lawyer originally from Green Lake, led the Masked Makers, a group of local seamstresses who sewed and distributed thousands of masks, featuring beautiful Indigenous designs, to children, elders, and home care workers.[4] Saskatchewan manufacturers switched their production to making face masks and shields, and distilleries started making hand sanitizer. People helped.

They helped as volunteers, as neighbours, and in jobs that changed right underneath them. Many people took on new ways of helping out during the COVID crisis. Others saw their jobs go from quiet, behind-the-scenes work to playing central roles in the daily unfolding drama of case updates, changing public health orders, and the dynamic interplay between political choices and public health advice.

Before this time, it's unlikely that most Canadian people could name the head of public health in their province. Now people like Dr. Tam, Deena Hinshaw in Alberta, and Robert Strang in Nova Scotia are household names across Canada. Bonnie Henry of British Columbia was featured in the *New York Times* and even had a pair of John Fluevog shoes designed in her honour.[5] They were put in positions of greater power and responsibility than any public health professionals in Canada's history, asked to advise and inform the public on how to safely go about their lives at a time when so much was dangerous and uncertain. Health promotion and disease prevention are what public health is always about, but these specialists found themselves under a spotlight they'd never imagined. With varying degrees of independence, they were forced to navigate not only the science of a rapidly spreading and changing infectious disease but also the demands of the public they served and the politicians who made the ultimate decisions on public health interventions. They were given credit when things went well, and sometimes blame when they did not, or when people didn't like the message.

In Saskatchewan, our fashion icon was known for knit sweaters, not fashionable shoes. Dr. Saqib Shahab, the province's chief medical health officer since 2012, was thrust into the spotlight as the face of our pandemic response. His regular press conferences, with him seated six feet away from the premier or the minister of health, became the source of key information, an object of admiration from the public, and the subject of great scrutiny throughout the COVID-19 crisis.

Born in Britain, Dr. Shahab studied medicine in Pakistan, later training in internal medicine in the United Kingdom and receiving his master's in public health from Johns Hopkins University in Baltimore. He completed his Royal College specialty training in public health at the University of Alberta before moving to practice in Yorkton, Saskatchewan, in 2001.[6]

Dr. Shahab is not the first in his family to find himself in the public eye. His father, Qudrut Ullah Shahab, was a high-ranking civil servant, first under the British Raj and eventually to the president in independent Pakistan. His autobiography, *Shahab Nama*, ranges from political commentary to mysticism and is one of the most celebrated books written in Urdu. He died the day Saqib graduated from Rawalpindi Medical College in Punjab province.[7]

In his early career, Dr. Shahab practised with a relief organization in Pakistan. He described this as the most exhilarating period of his career. Being in the middle of the action, even if the circumstances are stressful, is exhilarating and life-affirming. One wonders if some of that early career feeling returned for him during what he described as twenty-hour days at the beginning of the pandemic.

Along with those visible public figures were thousands of people whose ordinary jobs were no longer anything close to ordinary. Windows across Canada sported hearts for heroes, celebrating local health care workers as the heartbreaking stories from Italy and New York made it clear what the risks really were. The concept of essential workers was completely reimagined. Gas station attendants and grocery clerks, often low-paying entry-level employees, were being asked to risk their health to keep the rest of us whole. There was a sense of sacrifice, of stepping up to do what's right, and maybe, just maybe, a sense that that's what life is truly about.

In postwar North America, the people who had sacrificed so much for their country witnessed just what government can mobilize when the occasion demands and political will allows. That Greatest Generation insisted on the foundational programs we take for granted: Medicare, Old Age Security, publicly owned utilities, etc. But since the 1970s, that spirit of collective investment, of public ownership, of the commonwealth in its true meaning, has been steadily and deliberately eroded. Our country – and many countries around the world – seems to have lost the ability or the appetite to respond to great challenges, be they longer-term challenges of poverty and inequality, of changing health needs, or acute crises like that presented by COVID-19. Deliberate political decisions to undermine the very idea of the public good have left us weaker, sicker, poorer. The question before us now is whether this crisis, which demonstrated how important a force for good government can and must be, will revive the demand for better government that once coursed through Canada's political discourse.

The personal sacrifice and acts of "COVID kindness" we celebrated in those early days were the manifestation of a sense of connectedness and a desire for people to put their care into action. Alongside that feeling was a hope that awareness of the ways in which our individual well-being was dependent on the collective would result in wise choices, not just when it came to public health measures but also in the benefits extended to those most in need. And to some degree, that's exactly what happened. National programs like the Canada Emergency Response Benefit (CERB) and the Canada Emergency Wage Subsidy (CEWS) provided some standard support across the country for those who were unable to work and for businesses needing help paying wages while their ability to operate was greatly reduced or stopped altogether.

Each province came up with some measures of support as well, but this is where the idea of a nationwide effort falls apart. The Canadian response was provincial and patchwork and its effectiveness varied wildly from place to place and wave to wave. That first wave and the immediate quarantine period that accompanied it was perhaps the time when the experiences were most common. There were differences in the provincial responses, but they were of degree, not character as we would see in later waves. People and their families found something special in that shared experience of not having shared experiences. Most of us spent that unusually frozen March taking the calls to stay home seriously and trying to understand the changes happening around us.

Silent Spring

When I think of that spring of 2020, I'm in the little red house on Third Avenue that served as my constituency office the entire time I was the MLA for Saskatoon Meewasin. And I have an eight-year-old with me.

After the emergency end to the legislative session on March 18, I did the same as every other MLA, the same as so many people whose workplaces were no longer in person. I went home. I drove back to Saskatoon, where we entered the part of the pandemic that will stick with most of us the longest: those initial weeks of heavy quarantine. And I did what I could to make sure my own family was going to be okay. This meant keeping them safe and fed but also finding ways to make things fun for two little boys.

Mahli and I have two sons, Abraham and Augustin (Abe and Gus). At the time, Gus was two and Abe was eight. I went to the Safeway in my constituency and stocked up on pasta and canned goods, not knowing when we'd get back to a grocery store, and saw the shelves empty of toilet paper and Lysol wipes, of flour and sugar and baking powder. I recall hitting our local bookstore to load up on reading material for the whole family. Mahli and I indulged some of our doctor's gallows humour, playing the Pandemic board game, rereading Camus's *The Plague,* and making a somewhat tongue-in-cheek "staylist playlist"[8] on Spotify to share the songs that were getting us through. On that list were songs by John Prine, who lost his life to COVID on April 7. He'd been my favourite songwriter since my brother Jim brought a cassette tape of his music home to the farm when I was a kid. I'd grown up listening to and playing his songs, and his melancholic, quirky songwriting really did capture the feelings of that moment in many ways. I joined in the mourning by posting a cover of "Paradise," one of his many bittersweet songs about death. Prine was also the first of what would turn out to be very few legends or celebrities to die from COVID-19, which says a lot about how this, like so many other illnesses, affects those with privilege and wealth less than it does those whose lives are already hard. The social determinants are protective in the long term; material success helps to prevent many long-term illnesses like heart disease and diabetes. It also provides people with the means to safely and comfortably keep themselves away from illness and to seek testing and care when they need it.

With that in mind, I have to recognize how privileged we were during that time. Mahli could work in the hospital or do virtual clinics from her office. I could safely go to my constituency office to work. We had a child care plan for our kids. We didn't lose employment or pay. We didn't get sick. We were the lucky ones.

That winter was frigid and long, which may have helped people accept staying inside in those early quarantine times to slow the spread of the virus. But with schools and playgrounds and every indoor activity closed, we had to find some way to get out and live. On weekends we would pack Abe, Gus, and our dog, MG, into the car, pick a direction, and drive out of town. We would visit the famously strange Crooked Trees near Alticane, the Mount Carmel Shrine near Humboldt, and the Douglas Provincial Park sand dunes, or just get drive-through and find a random field to run around and let off some steam.

During the week, not a lot changed for Gus. With me away so much in Regina and Mahli busy in her practice, we'd had someone coming to the house to help with Gus since Mahli finished her maternity leave. That arrangement continued, with some trepidation as we were limiting every contact we could, but it would have been impossible for us to continue our work without that help.

As for Abe, he hung out with me. Each morning we would head into my MLA office. When the weather warmed up, we would pedal our bikes through an eerily deserted downtown Saskatoon. With schools having closed so quickly, teachers hadn't had time to adapt seriously to online learning, so the end of Grade 3 consisted of an hour or so of online school every morning, and then office time with Dad. The first several sessions of this were pretty comical, as the teachers scrambled to learn the tech while the kids, all digital natives, went wild in the chat section. Eventually, they settled down to a routine with daily homework, keeping some learning going and alleviating some of Abe's boredom. After his classes, Abe would read Percy Jackson books or play on the iPad (full disclosure: his screen time limits expanded as well) while I tried to keep doing my province-wide job from one small space.

Like everyone, our opposition team had to figure out how to communicate while being unable to gather. I would hold daily press conferences and put out videos speaking directly to the people of Saskatchewan about the latest developments in our knowledge of the virus or our latest call for government action to respond to the economic and health disaster.

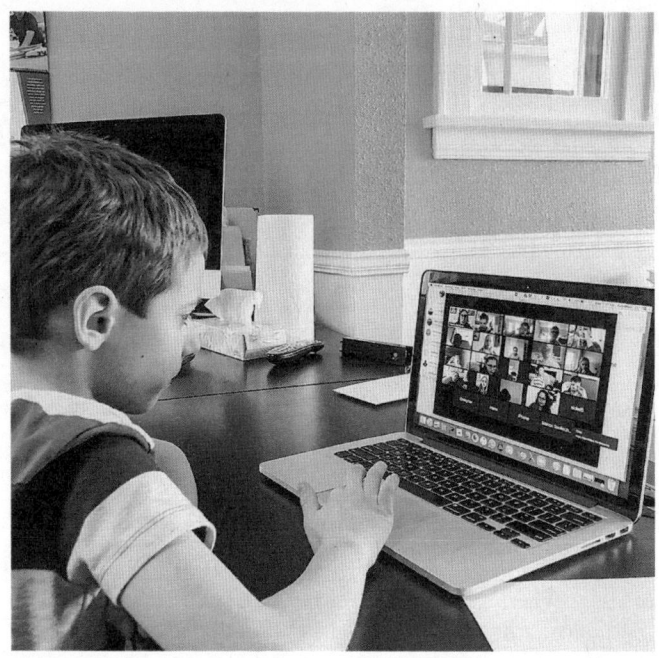

Abe attends school remotely from the MLA office. April 2020

Using platforms like Zoom or YouTube, Facebook Live or Microsoft Teams seems second nature now, but it took a while for us to figure out our end and reporters to figure out theirs. I would set up my laptop and microphone on top of a stack of chairs and cardboard boxes, trying to get the angle and sound just right, and hope we didn't get too many tech failures. I spent so much time in online meetings those first few weeks that I wound up needing the glasses I now refer to as my "zoom lenses." I am in my mid-forties, so it's not entirely surprising, but it was a noticeable change. We released regular calls for action from a government that, while no longer dismissing the threat of COVID-19 outright, was still slow to act, especially when it came to supporting frontline workers and the most vulnerable.

Abe and I would stop and have lunch together then pedal back home after a few more hours of work. We've always been close, but as much as this time was stressful, there was a sweetness to it, something special about being forced to be just the two of us for long days. When I think

First Wave

back to those times, I have to confess to some nostalgia. For all the risk and responsibility we felt and the fear we shared with those around us, being hunkered down with the kids was special. We connected on what was important in ways we'll never forget.

Spreading the Word

Fortunately for us all, COVID-19 hit Saskatchewan later than other parts of Canada, and – through interprovincial peer and public pressure – the province introduced public health measures at about the same time. This meant that the first wave in Saskatchewan, while not insignificant – nothing that makes people sick and takes human lives should be treated as insignificant – was nowhere near as bad as it could have been, nowhere near as bad as many parts of Canada.

All in all, we tried to bring people a balance of serious concern and hope amid dire warnings. A document leaked from the SHA showed modelling saying that, without major public health measures, 30 percent of the population could contract COVID, leading to deaths of up to 15,000 people in our province of just over a million.[9] This would prove, thanks to behaviour changes, changes in the virus, the eventual arrival of vaccination, and improvements in modelling, to be a great overestimate of what did happen. It's a classic example of the paradox of preparation:[10] if the measures taken work and nothing bad happens, then you must have overreacted. These initial models of the extreme scenario without measures in place led to measures being put in place. The fact that the modelling overshot what went on to occur is a feature, not a bug. This is a public health victory, and a public action victory. The vast majority of Canadians heard the call to safety and listened, many changing their behaviour dramatically, including maintaining small bubbles for all of the next two years.

Unfortunately, as modelling got more precise and more responsive to on-the-ground situations, people who knew better would disingenuously point to this early example to discredit that later modelling. We had what would later prove to be an extremely reliable and – had it been used properly – helpful tool for real-time response to changing community transmission and risk levels. Instead, we would see modelling become tragically accurate in subsequent phases because it was kept hidden rather than used to influence behaviour. Before any of this would play out, what we had before us at the end of March 2020 were credible indicators that a human health disaster was headed our way.

I remember very vividly sitting with Mahli, who is a general pediatrician, as we talked through what we would do. She works regularly in the hospital, and I had just renewed my licence to be able to step up as part of the medical team. Sitting on the sidelines was never an option; if we were needed, we would help. With the number of Italian doctors who died in that country's brutal first outbreak firmly in our minds,[11] we were making sure our wills were in order and talking through a plan for who would take Abe and Gus if we needed to go full-time into dangerous work, or worse, if we didn't come back. Our friends and colleagues in health care were all going through the same process, ready and willing to get to work, but also fully aware that this was uncharted and dangerous territory.

It was a scary time for everyone, but particularly confusing for kids, suddenly out of all their normal routines and hearing about a mysterious new malady. Given our young family and our professions, Mahli and I were particularly concerned with how kids would cope. On March 23, inspired by Erna Solberg, then prime minister of Norway, I hosted a press conference for Saskatchewan children. Kids from across the province sent in questions on what a virus is, whether trees and pets could catch COVID, why they couldn't visit their grandparents, whether their asthma made them higher risk, why their favourite sports were cancelled, why they couldn't play at the playground, and whether all the countries were working together on a cure for COVID. I did my best to respond honestly and in language that gave kids a sense of hope and agency, giving them tips on what they could do to keep their family safe and to help make life lighter for those around them.

Thinking back to those darkest early days of March 2020, it seems both like a lifetime ago and like we're still sorting through the debris of that initial shock and all the waves that followed. Often a great change means you're uprooted, displaced, like the refugees who have come here in recent years from Syria, Myanmar, or South Sudan. Instead, the pandemic made people refugees at home, sheltering in place. What that home was like, whether it was a safe place with supportive family or somewhere that was lonely, dangerous, or just plain poor, made a huge difference in your view of the pandemic. And of course, whether you were able to work from home, out working in the community because your job is an essential service, or out of work altogether put everything in a different light. But no matter what your circumstances, your world got smaller, just as the challenges got bigger. That disruption has caused fractures in our society that will take a very long time to heal – that is, for those of us who are still here.

Losing Trust

Alice Grove grew up on the farm east of North Battleford, the eldest of five children. In the 1970s she worked as a nurse's aide at the Saskatchewan Hospital, a large psychiatric facility in North Battleford, and later at the Riverside Seniors Home. She then farmed with her husband, Bruce, south of town until he passed away in 2004.

Alice and Bruce didn't have children, but she was very close with her younger sister, Eleanor Widdowson, and treated her sister's children and grandchildren like her own. A gifted musician, she played piano, accordion, and organ, clarinet in the Kinsmen Band, and bagpipes with the Battleford Legion Pipes and Drums. She loved to knit and crochet, especially making mittens and socks for children for church charity drives. She hosted yarn-spinning demonstrations at the Western Development Museum for nearly thirty years.

At seventy-five, what Alice enjoyed most was going into North Battleford to do her shopping and visit with friends. In early March 2020, Eleanor took Alice and a friend for coffee at the Walmart McDonald's. Eleanor told Alice that there was COVID around and she should stay home, that she'd bring her groceries out to the farm and come visit. Alice insisted on coming into town; there were no local cases being reported and she was lonely on the farm.

Two weeks later, Eleanor was just home from her shift in food services at the new Saskatchewan Hospital when she got a call that Alice had collapsed at home and been rushed to the Battlefords Union Hospital.

She'd required ventilator support to keep breathing. The next morning Eleanor got a call that her sister wasn't doing well and she should come to the hospital right away.

Eleanor knew Alice wasn't in shape to fight through COVID pneumonia. She had underlying lung disease and had also been diabetic for years, with resulting kidney and heart troubles. She was exactly the sort of person we were flattening the curve for, someone who needed to be kept safe until a vaccine or treatment was available because there was no way she could survive infection without that protection. That morning, as Alice's oxygen saturation dropped from the high eighties to the low fifties, Eleanor realized it was the end. She sat with her daughter and watched the monitors through the window of the ICU, unable to go in and say goodbye.

At 8:21 a.m. on Saturday, March 28, 2020, Alice became the first Saskatchewan person to die from COVID-19. The original death certificate did not include COVID-19 as a diagnosis, as the test wouldn't be positive until the next day. This gives some insight into how deaths that happened before a final diagnosis or happened outside hospital might not end up being included in the official tally of COVID fatalities.

When Eleanor insisted that the certificate be changed to include COVID the next day, she met resistance until she threatened to demand an autopsy. She felt things were being hidden from the public and became even more frustrated when she went to work that Monday and learned there were still no reported deaths from COVID in the province. That's when she decided to take her story to the media because she believed that the government "should be telling where people are dying." She decided that even if the government didn't want to say what had happened to her sister, she had to. She wanted Alice's death to be a warning to others, and she wanted to call for greater transparency.

Eleanor took the lesson from her sister's illness very seriously. When we spoke in the fall of 2022, she'd had her initial vaccine series and two boosters and had so far steered clear of COVID. She's happy she's been able to stay healthy, but still misses her sister. Sometimes she forgets Alice is gone and thinks of giving her a call.

As she speaks about her sister, the old frustration returns. At that time, case counts were still being announced with very little localizing information. Locations of deaths would not be included in reporting until mid-April. Eleanor believes the province missed an opportunity, that if it had been more transparent, identifying that there were cases in North Battleford, Alice and other seniors might have been more cautious. She says that "it shouldn't have happened. If the government had been a little less secretive, maybe it wouldn't have. If something else comes along in the future, I hope they won't be pulling stuff like that. People need to know."

This was one of the major failings of an otherwise robust early pandemic response, and though it would change over time, limiting information would be a constant theme throughout the pandemic. In a late 2020 article, despite being in the midst of a punishing and deadly second wave, Scott Moe said he wouldn't change a thing about his response so far. In that article, he reported receiving the following advice from his predecessor, Brad Wall: "Just never lose your gut instincts on where people are, and how people want to be treated, and what they want to hear."[1] In response to the falsehoods being propagated concerning the outcome of the 2020 US election, Oklahoma City mayor David Holt wrote that "the greatest, most dangerous, and most frequent temptation faced by an elected official is the temptation to tell your constituents what they want to hear."[2] From the very beginning of the COVID-19 pandemic in Saskatchewan, we saw that philosophy on full display, with downplaying of the seriousness of the health and economic challenges a constant and increasing feature of the province's public pronouncements. The worst manifestation of this would be the decision in early 2022 to reduce overall access to testing and to greatly reduce the frequency of public reporting, going from daily updates to weekly and then monthly data dumps, but the instinct to limit information was there from the beginning.

There are two ways that limiting information weakened our ability to successfully motivate the public. First, the lack of official information gave more space to misinformation as people turned to less reliable sources. More insidiously, the lack of trust in the public, demonstrated by the government's decision to limit information, was reciprocated by a loss of trust in those official sources. Even when the news is bad, more news is better. A study of 177 countries in the *Lancet* showed that the places that had the highest level of trust in their government had the lowest rates of infection and highest rates of vaccination.[3] When you trust others with the truth, they are more likely to trust you. When you downplay the seriousness of a situation and try to spin everything as a good news story, the eventual reckoning with reality erodes the trust and goodwill in public institutions and expert opinion needed in times of crisis.

I won't pretend that I have never taken the option of trying to tell people what I thought they wanted to hear. It's never admirable, but it's a temptation we all succumb to at times. It's also a constant debate in political backrooms: How much do you lead people with strong positions versus how much do you follow the estimation of what people are ready for that's provided by opinion polling? That spring, however, the stakes seemed too high to wait for people to be ready for reality. What was needed was leadership willing to say the hard things.

Calls to Action

In those early days, I kept up as much video information sharing as I could. There was a need for straight, clear talk, for a calm, rational voice between the poles of panic and passivity, amidst all the confusing and often conflicting information coming from official sources and social media. This led me to do something a bit unusual for a politician: post a video on how to make your own masks. Most of us who have now gone through boxes and boxes of disposable face masks had never worn a mask of any kind before, outside of Halloween. Even as a doctor, I hadn't worn one since med school except when assisting in the operating room for the occasional C-section. And while cloth masks are not as effective as standard medical masks, which aren't as effective as N95 respirator-style masks, they still provide a level of protection.

Initially, Canadian public health leadership resisted recommending widespread mask use.[4] Along with slowness in identifying that SARS-CoV-2 was airborne and accepting masks as an effective method of preventing transmission, some of the reluctance was rooted in the scarcity of personal protective equipment (PPE) materials. At the time medical masks were not widely available and there were legitimate worries about seeing hospital-grade masks diverted to public use. As the evidence for mask use grew, I took a cue from the #Masks4All movement out of Czechia and decided to promote the use of homemade cloth masks.[5] On April 5, I filmed a video at home on how to make an effective if not beautiful simple cloth mask with scissors, cloth, and a paper towel filter.[6]

At first, I got some questioning on why I was jumping ahead, recommending masks when public health wasn't. Then the next day, after having recommended against masks throughout March, Dr. Theresa Tam changed course and joined the US Centers for Disease Control and Prevention (CDC) in recommending masks.[7] Saskatchewan wouldn't see an official recommendation until the end of May. Scott Moe wouldn't put one on until late July, after even Donald Trump had appeared in public with a mask. This reluctance from the top to encourage the use of masks helped fuel the anti-mask rhetoric that was already taking root in Saskatchewan in the summer of 2020 and would later shift to promotion of ineffective medications like Ivermectin and anti-vaccine misinformation. It's a shame that masks, a simple and non-intrusive intervention that could allow us to safely carry on so much of our daily lives even before the arrival of vaccines, became so controversial. As our understanding of their effectiveness and the availability of masks improved, they could have been a symbol of the solidarity that had characterized the early days of the pandemic. Instead, they became a partisan wedge, with people judging each other's deeper world views by whether or not they had a piece of fabric on their face.

Along with this direct outreach and information sharing with the public, our opposition team looked to be a voice for what positive measures could be taken to support people in a challenging time. We also continued to seek opportunities to collaborate across party lines. I wrote to the premier offering to help and encouraging him to

establish a special committee to provide guidance and direction for the government's response to the COVID-19 pandemic. That committee should include members from the Government and the Official Opposition Caucuses, along with leaders from all over the province – including First Nations and Metis, municipal leaders, leaders in key sectors such as health, education, social services and justice, and business and labour leaders – to address both the immediate health crisis and the economic impacts going forward.[8]

Sadly, this sincere offer was rejected as well.

In the absence of a chance to do so around a common table, we continued to speak through the media to call for necessary public health measures, action on health system readiness, cooperation with municipal and First Nations leaders, and supports for people who were out of work or having a hard time. Often, the government would turn around and do these things a few days later, other times our advice and the examples of other jurisdictions would go unheeded.

The one area where the Sask Party seemed particularly reluctant to help was in supports for the most vulnerable. They were very reluctant to agree to a moratorium on evictions, even though it made no sense for people who were being told to stay home to be kicked out of their homes. Along with those at risk for becoming homeless, there was an urgent need to help those already homeless or in precarious housing. Shelters had to reduce the number of beds they were opening, and community agencies had their doors closed. People had nowhere to go and were at the mercy of the weather and the virus. Eventually we were able to push the minister of justice to stop evictions. Added supports for food security or the organizations serving homeless people never did appear.

The Saskatoon Inter-Agency Response team, a group of community organizations working in the city's core neighbourhoods, released a comparison of different supports across Canada.[9] Quebec had opened 541 new housing units and dedicated $30 million in new funding. In Ontario there were 2,126 new units and $200 million dollars, 142 units and $1.2 million in Manitoba. Alberta had made 498 new units available and dedicated $30 million, and British Columbia made the largest investment, with 900 housing units and $1.2 billion in new funding. These provinces had recognized the need to make extra investments in those at risk, in addition to the CERB funding of $500 per month from the federal government for those eligible. In Saskatchewan, a grand total of $171,000 was distributed among ten housing initiatives for cleaning supplies and only 10 new housing units were made available. Social assistance recipients received a one-time top-up of $50, but also saw CERB payments clawed back from their social assistance cheques.[10] For reasons that are hard to fathom at any time, but particularly at a time when so many were struggling, the Sask Party preferred that additional federal dollars flow into provincial coffers rather than stay with people living in poverty.

Dusting Off the Stethoscope

For me, there was never any question. As soon as we knew there would be an added need, it was obvious that Mahli and I would be willing to pitch in. It's why we went into medicine in the first place and, while the shape of that commitment changes with family roles, age, patterns of illness, personal interests, etc., that core drive to help the sick never goes away.

On March 13 I applied for an emergency licence through the College of Physicians and Surgeons, having stopped active medical practice shortly after becoming leader of the NDP in the spring of 2018. After getting my licence and practice privileges, I signed up to work at a COVID-19 testing and assessment site and do weekly clinics at the Lighthouse emergency shelter and supported living home in downtown Saskatoon. In April I joined a team at the Core Neighbourhood testing site in the gym at Princess Alexandra School. The sites were run by public health and a team of docs, nurses, social workers, and administrative staff. This was where people were sent who had COVID symptoms or exposure and needed not only testing but also a medical assessment. This was my first experience with something all health care workers would get very used to: donning and doffing of full PPE. Getting the sequence of putting on gowns and gloves and face masks, serial hand sanitizing, and handling the samples safely took some getting used to but was so important for not getting sick or spreading the virus to others. The staff at the testing site were incredibly dedicated and professional and helped me to immediately feel a part of the team.

At the time, case numbers were low and so was test demand. Some days we had people coming in with significant medical and social issues. A couple of times we jumped in our vehicles in full PPE and went out to people's homes for testing and medical care, or to the hotel where people who had tested positive but didn't have a safe home to isolate in were staying. This felt strangely adventurous, as though we were out after curfew even though it was the middle of the day. On other days, we had more staff than patients. This might be seen as a failure but adding extra testing and tracing capacity was the smart thing to do. The big failure wasn't excess capacity in the beginning; it was decreasing that capacity in the months to follow rather than building it up when it was clear a second wave was on the way. The "efficient" choice meant that the essential role of testing and tracing in identifying and controlling outbreaks was never as effective as it should have been.

At the Lighthouse, Jeannie Coe and her team of nurse practitioners run daily clinics serving the residents, working alongside an incredible group of outreach workers, front staff, case managers, cooks, home care workers, and addictions counsellors. The Lighthouse has been operating since the 1990s in the former Capri hotel and serves a clientele of people who are at various stages of struggles with trauma, substance abuse and addiction, mental illness, and deep poverty. It is a place that knows violence, anguish, despair, and also kindness, humour, and solidarity. The presence of the largest homeless shelter in the province in its largest city's downtown core has been a source of repeated controversy. Whether or not downtown is the ideal place for the Lighthouse, it is frustrating that the nuisance of its location bothers people more than the fact that such a facility is needed in a province as wealthy as ours.

For me, while I hadn't worked at the Lighthouse itself before, it was a homecoming of sorts. Many of the residents there are also patients at West Side Community Clinic, where I'd worked before getting elected. In a way, it was even more interesting to see them at home and surrounded by supports. Not that things are always smooth; people don't wind up staying at the Lighthouse because they've had easy lives. Childhood trauma, mental illness, and substance use disorders are the norm, along with frequently severe medical or post-traumatic disability. People can be stable and steady for months on end, and then "decompensate," meaning they need much more intense care. Others are permanently on the edge of returning to the street, needing in-patient care, or winding up in jail. There have been some changes at the Lighthouse in recent months due to management issues, but up to that point the facility hosted direct housing supports for people living in two housing towers, a managed alcohol harm reduction program, a stabilization unit for those who were still using and on the street, and numerous other programs to help people who were dealing with a complex web of trauma, substance abuse, mental illness, and poverty.

People experiencing homelessness and shelter populations always face a higher risk of illness. Dr. Naheed Dosani, who founded the Palliative Education and Care for the Homeless (PEACH) program in Toronto,[11] has described homelessness as a "terminal illness"[12] given the dramatically shortened life expectancy of those living on the streets. COVID offered a new risk and a different challenge. Given the complexity of street and shelter life, one of the big worries was that physical distancing just wouldn't be possible. Add to that complex underlying medical conditions, illnesses like COPD, HIV, heart disease, diabetes, and more, and the people at the Lighthouse and other shelters were extremely high-risk. One early report described how "among the most vulnerable to the virus, people who are experiencing homelessness are 20 times more likely to be hospitalized for COVID-19, 10 times more likely to receive intensive care, and more than five times more likely to die within 21 days of a positive test."[13] With COVID-19 further highlighting the danger that lack of housing puts people in, perhaps we will finally have the conversation about why a country this wealthy is comfortable seeing ever-increasing numbers of people without safe and secure housing.

Shortly after renewing my licence, I got in touch with Jeannie to see if I could come and volunteer at the Lighthouse. She and her team made me feel immediately welcome and I started going in on Friday mornings. For the next two years I got to know the residents and the staff that worked so hard to support them. They put in a tremendous effort to encourage the residents and clients to use masks and hand sanitizer, to protect themselves and avoid outbreaks. I remember my heart sinking when, on a break from clinics during the election, I got a text from Jeannie telling me there was an outbreak of dozens of cases at the Lighthouse.[14] Very few became seriously ill that time, but that luck wouldn't hold. There would be multiple other outbreaks and a number of residents would wind up in hospital or die from COVID in the following year.

I felt a sense of duty to return to work, for sure. I also got an incredible amount of joy from those Friday clinics. They were my break from the big picture. The COVID-19 pandemic was a massive, all-consuming event. It was disorienting and frightening for everyone, myself included. At the same time, as it brought back idealistic youthful feelings of abandoning one's own interests to serve the health of others, of being able to pitch in to help with a bigger cause, seeing patients helped to order one corner of the swirling storm. I was reminded why I became a doctor and why I got into politics. The return to practice and the chance to be part of the conversation about the larger response gave me a sense of purpose in a confusing time. I can't help but think that the lack of such an outlet for so many, the lack of agency, the powerlessness, helped to feed some of the dysfunction that would follow.

Reopening Minds

On April 23, 2020, forty days after introducing a state of emergency, Scott Moe declared that Saskatchewan had "flattened the curve" and announced his Re-Open Saskatchewan plan in a live television address.[1] By mid-April, we were seeing single-digit new cases of COVID-19 and our case counts and hospitalizations were among the lowest in the country.[2]

Saskatchewan has less international travel than major hubs like Toronto, Vancouver, and Montreal, meaning our first cases arrived later. As other provinces took action, the peer pressure of the moment forced our government to act as well. This meant we had the good luck of seeing our first cases arrive at the same time as public health measures were brought in. New cases spiked briefly, largely from returning travellers, but the stringent measures and high level of concern from Saskatchewan people kept that spread to a minimum. Those who could had stayed home, others had gone to work on the frontlines to make sure people had what they needed. People had reached out to help their neighbours and their communities. We were flattening the curve and it was a remarkable achievement that allowed us to enjoy a window of relief from the intensity of the first wave.

Because of the life cycle of a circulating virus and the seasonal nature of human interactions, COVID risk waxes and wanes. The mistake wasn't lifting COVID restrictions when things got better; it was failing to say they would likely be back. Allowing people to enjoy life more during safer times is sensible and necessary for them to get the respite they need.

What is dangerous is the establishment of a false sense of security or finality. If future restrictions are necessary, people will be more able to accept them if they've had a break, but only if the possibility of a return is signalled in advance. Instead, we've seen each abatement of the virus be described as the end of the pandemic, only to repeat the same errors with subsequent waves. It's as though each spring we burned our parkas and declared that winter would never return. Summer gets us through winter; knowing winter will be back makes us enjoy summer even more.

Dancing Lessons

In his March 2020 article "The Hammer and the Dance," Tomas Pueyo described a viral suppression approach to flattening the curve. The first step is the hammer: "First, you act quickly and aggressively ... We want to quench this thing as soon as possible."[3] By introducing effective measures quickly, you stop the virus before it spreads widely. Then comes the tricky part: "a dance of measures between getting our lives back on track and spreading the disease."[4] There are specifics to the dance: the surveillance methods of testing and tracing that help to identify whether we're in a high- or low-risk window, the first measures to bring in, the first to relax, what rates of transmission should trigger measures, etc.

During the first two years of the pandemic, before Omicron and immunity changed the game, we could watch examples around the world of places that did the dance well, enduring brief periods of serious measures in order to enjoy longer windows of more normal life. Among Organisation for Economic Co-operation and Development (OECD) countries, Japan and New Zealand had the lowest death rates per capita.[5] Japan also has the highest percentage of elderly residents, making this an even more notable accomplishment. Major restrictions were not in place for much of the pandemic, but there was high social buy-in for masking and social distancing, widespread acceptance of vaccination, and a robust public health system that was effective in testing and tracing, all of which kept COVID transmission under control.[6] In New Zealand, more severe restrictions on travel, schools, and businesses were put in place as part of a proactive elimination approach. This resulted in death rates a quarter of what was experienced in Canada, and longer periods without restrictions as low levels of circulating virus allowed for quicker and longer-lasting reopenings than places that had to shut down once the virus was already circulating widely.[7]

Closer to home, the experience of the "Atlantic Bubble" saw the provinces of Eastern Canada take a suppression approach rather than mitigation, and as a result they have lower case and fatality rates than their Western counterparts, along with shorter periods of economically and socially restrictive public health measures. If our disjointed national response was a natural experiment, the East was the intervention group, the Prairies were the control.

In Saskatchewan and Alberta, like most of the United States, each time case numbers improved, the message people received wasn't, "Thank you for your sacrifices; because of them we've done well and are better prepared for the next wave"; it was, "Too much has been asked of you, it is all over now." The latter message set us up for failure in later waves, as people simply weren't psychologically prepared to return to a phase they'd been told they could leave behind. You heard people saying things like, "We were told it would be a couple of weeks," as though COVID had broken a promise. They weren't wrong, but that promise was made by politicians. The virus wouldn't listen to lawmakers. People underestimated both the luck and the effort it took to enjoy that early success, and this would come back to haunt us as we headed into subsequent waves, as people had come to believe that it "couldn't happen here." In the summer of 2020, comparing ourselves with places like Ontario and Quebec, which had to call in the military, or with places like Spain that had declared states of emergency, Saskatchewan seemed like it had weathered the storm. What we failed to do was prepare for the storms to come.

Scott Moe's 2020 reopening plan was largely sensible. There was room for criticism as businesses being asked to reopen wondered where they would get the PPE needed to do so, and quibbles about how the province had managed to prioritize opening golf courses but kept kids' playgrounds closed. Still, there was a spirit of willingness to fumble through these complicated changes together. Given the optimism and pride people were feeling at how well things had gone in the province thus far, I saw no need to pick the plan apart. Instead, I reminded the government that there were still people who needed help. In Alberta, Ontario, and British Columbia, there were investments of $400 to $600 per person in provincial supports. In Saskatchewan, that number was less than $60.[8] With thousands of jobs lost, with businesses having closed their doors and uncertain whether they would successfully open them again, with frontline workers making the country's lowest minimum wage, this was not the time to declare victory and leave people to their own devices.

The main problem with the reopening plan was not one of policy but of tense. By saying we had flattened the curve, the impression Moe gave was not that we were in a window, but rather that we were looking at something in our rear-view mirror. In that vehicle, there was a gas pedal and forward gears, but no brakes and no reverse. The delicate dance of relaxing and reintroducing restrictions needed to be communicated and laid out in the plan. For example: if we reach a certain number of cases or hospitalizations, we'll have to return to Phase 1; if the rate of spread increases by a certain amount, we'll have to introduce mandatory masking. If we get to point A, we can relax; if we get to point B, we tighten up. This approach has risk because it means you commit ahead of time but need to have the humility to say the future isn't certain. On the other hand, it allows for greater transparency, permitting a government to be more honest with people about the limitations of their knowledge and perhaps setting the stage for a public that is more prepared to deal with ambiguity and change.

Northern Exposure

In late April, a worker returning home from Fort McMurray, Alberta, passed the virus on to a family member who worked in long-term care in the Northwest community of La Loche. COVID then spread quickly through the combined hospital and long-term care home, the town, and the neighbouring on-reserve community of Clearwater River Dene Nation. This would be hard on any community, but La Loche is a place that has experienced an incredible amount of tragedy and grief. Just a couple of months earlier had been the four-year anniversary of the devastating school shooting at Dene High. By the time the outbreak was declared over in July, nearly 300 people had tested positive and 5 had died in what was the largest outbreak in an Indigenous community to that point.[9] What prevented it from being far worse was the work of local leaders who organized temporary housing for isolation, set up food distribution, and hosted fifty SHA workers who came into the community for aggressive testing and tracing of positive cases.

For months prior, Northern and on-reserve communities had been setting up checkpoints in their communities and asking the government for support to control who went in and out. Local leaders set up the 155 Collective – referring to Highway 155, which serves the Northwest from Green Lake to La Loche – organizing food distribution, information sharing, and community supports during the most serious periods of lockdown.[10] During medical school and into the early years of practice, I had spent a lot of time in Northern Saskatchewan, including in La Loche. I was familiar with the strengths of local communities, the incredible Dene, Cree, and Métis cultures, and the beauty of the immense forests and myriad lakes. I was also aware, as were local leaders, that the social challenges of the North were significant. Mayors and Chiefs recognized that overcrowded housing, high rates of underlying illness, and behaviours associated with substance abuse helped create the conditions for quick spread and deadly outcomes. The La Loche outbreak confirmed those fears.

The province, after having refused to discuss closing communities with those that requested it and even prioritizing access to recreational properties for people from the South, decided to lock down the entire North. Now it wasn't outsiders unable to come in: locals weren't allowed to leave. People were fined for driving south to get groceries. Northerners who had to attend medical appointments in the South reported facing discrimination.

Dr. Kendra Morrow, a Saskatoon family doctor, teamed up with a group of medical students from the University of Saskatchewan to raise nearly $50,000 in donations for La Loche. The group worked with local trucking companies to send food, drinking water, toys, and cleaning supplies.[11] To help support this effort, a friend and I filled a half-ton with meat and fresh vegetables donated by local food suppliers and hand sanitizer we'd sourced from one of the local distilleries. We drove it as far as the checkpoint at Green Lake, parking at the Keewatin junction and transferring the supplies into the pickup of one of the 155 Collective volunteers. We saw the incredible resourcefulness of the local leadership, but also heard the frustration. As one of the volunteers said to me, "They weren't interested in helping us keep COVID out, but now that it's here they're happy to keep us in." This pattern of ignoring the North until it was too late would continue, most seriously when Moe blamed hard-hit communities for the fourth wave.[12]

Walking With Our Angels

That summer window also saw a summer of protest. Perhaps, as some have suggested, the sense of isolation had people searching for community action.[13] The murder of George Floyd in Minnesota had led to Black Lives Matter protests all over the world, including a thousand-strong march in downtown Saskatoon. We also saw the emergence of anti-mask protests locally.[14] These would start with a dozen or so people but grow and shift over the coming months to be part of an increasingly influential movement.

Unique to Saskatchewan was a protest of a different sort. Tristen Durocher is an accomplished Métis fiddle player from Buffalo Narrows. He speaks quietly, often with a mysterious smile, but beneath that gentleness is a hard confidence. He knows what he believes and is not afraid to tell you. In the summer of 2020, he was sick of playing his fiddle at funerals for people younger than him.

Saskatchewan has the highest rate of suicide in the country, double the national average, with over 2,200 people dying by suicide in the last fifteen years. Thousands more have attempted to end their lives. This number is shocking enough, but it can obscure the fact that a large percentage of these premature deaths are happening to young people in the North. A First Nations boy in Saskatchewan is six times more likely to lose his life by suicide than other children in the province. For First Nations girls, that number rises to thirty.[15] An enormous region, nearly half the land that makes up the province, Northern Saskatchewan is home to only about 40,000 people. The historical trauma of residential schools and colonization is compounded by the contemporary grief of poverty and loss. With young people in the North dying by suicide at a rate far higher than the rest of the province, every community, every family has been touched by suicide.

Doyle Vermette is the NDP MLA for Cumberland, covering Northeast Saskatchewan. He has spent years counselling families to try to prevent suicide and consoling those who have lost loved ones, and he brings the pain of those families to his work in the legislature. In 2018, he recognized that, despite those leading statistics, Saskatchewan does not have a suicide prevention strategy. Well-designed strategies can have an enormous impact, as demonstrated in Quebec, where the overall suicide rate fell by 30 percent and the youth suicide rate by 50 percent in the years following the introduction of a strategy.[16] Doyle worked with grieving families and leaders in mental health to prepare a private member's bill to try to change that. The Saskatchewan Party government let Doyle's bill die on the Order Paper in 2019, making Saskatchewan the only place in the country to see a motion for suicide prevention not be unanimously proclaimed, let alone defeated.[17] Instead the government released Pillars for Life,[18] a document described by Jack Hicks, an expert in suicide prevention, as "so vague as to be meaningless."[19]

We introduced the bill a second time, and Doyle continued to share the stories of those who were hurting. In November 2019, Chief Ronald Mitsuing of the Makwa Sahgaiehcan First Nation declared a state of crisis and emergency in his community after three suicides in three weeks, including of a ten-year-old girl, were followed by multiple attempts.[20] Mitsuing came to the legislature to plead with the government for action.

The tragedies kept coming. In May 2020, twenty-year-old football player Samwel Uko went twice to a Regina emergency room in a state of mental health crisis. Video would later show him screaming for help and being removed from the ER by hospital staff. He took his life later that afternoon, drowning in Wascana Lake.[21] His uncle, Justin Nyee, also joined in the call for a suicide prevention strategy, along with an inquiry into Samwel's death.[22]

It's hard to believe anyone could hear those stories and not want to act, but the government chose to vote against the bill at the end of June. Our opposition caucus had made this our priority bill for 2020, meaning it was the one bill we could force the government to vote on. On the last day of session, Scott Moe and his ministers listened intently to Doyle's passionate speech. They listened as he said that if this were happening in a community of 40,000 people in the South, in a community like my hometown of Moose Jaw, then we would see action. They listened as he spoke of the funerals he has had to attend. They listened to him pour his heart out and ask for so little, just the support for a bill that would make a difference. They nodded along, their hearts in their eyes. They even clapped for him when he finished. And then forty-four MLAs, every single member of the government caucus, including the premier and the cabinet, stood up and voted no.

Tristen Durocher was twenty-four and living in La Ronge at the time, back in Saskatchewan after COVID had ended his job teaching fiddle in Northern Manitoba schools. During those early days of COVID-19, he was reading a lot and following the news more closely. He saw people struggling more with mental health problems, saw people's addictions taking over in the aimless time of quarantine. When he heard about the government's rejection of Doyle's bill, he thought of all those who had been lost in his community and around the province, and he decided he needed to do something. With news coming so fast, he didn't want this to be a one-day story; he wanted to keep the focus on the lives being lost. He wanted to make a difference.

Tristen consulted with Elders and then, along with Chris Merasty of Men of the North – a mental health support group based in La Ronge – began the Walking With Our Angels ceremony, a 635-kilometre walk from La Ronge to the Legislative Building. Once they arrived in Regina, Tristen planned to camp in Wascana Park across from the legislature and fast for forty-four days, one for each of the Sask Party MLAs who had voted against Doyle's bill.

A few days after their walk began, my son Abe and I met up with Tristen and Chris a few kilometres north of Prince Albert. They had a team of family members and friends supporting them, taking turns riding behind or walking alongside. We walked with the group into the city, where they were met with honks and people waving from the street. Both Tristen and Chris were welcoming and positive, knowing that what they were talking about was heavy, but wanting to give people a sense of

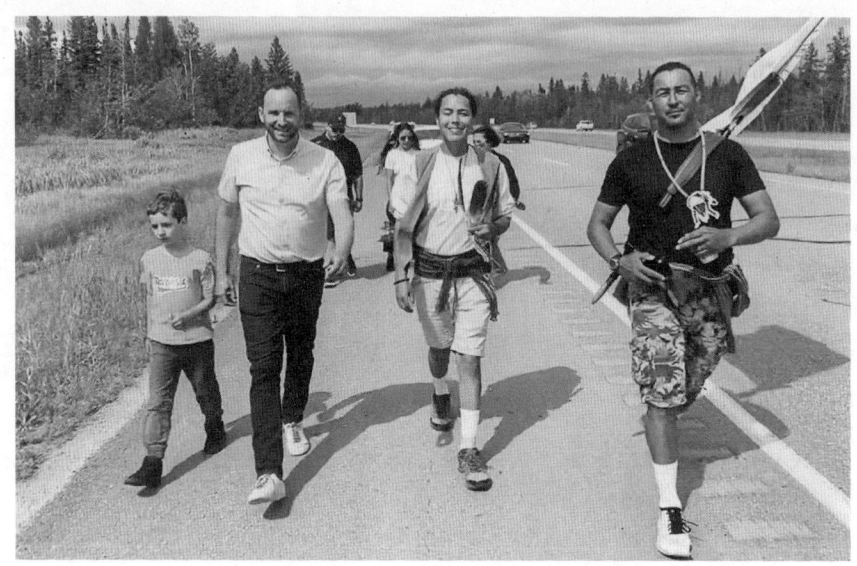

**Outside Prince Albert with Tristen Durocher and Chris Merasty
of the Walking With Our Angels ceremony. July 2020**

hope. We met with them again for the walk into Saskatoon, where my
friend James Sylvestre from the Buffalo River Dene Nation led drumming
and sacred songs. We then took part in a sharing circle, followed by
Tristen showing us why he's such a well-known fiddle player, with a
moving concert of traditional fiddle tunes.

On July 31, nearly a month after they'd left La Ronge, Walking With
Our Angels walked – tired, skinny, and sore but in high spirits – into
Regina. They marched up the steps of the legislature and presented prayers, a fiddle performance by Tristen, and a banner with the names of
those who had been lost to suicide. The group then proceeded to erect
a tepee in the park and to place photos of people lost to suicide, mounted
on wire and stuck into the grass, as a portrait gallery of whom they were
there to represent. Tristen made a point of saying that, while Indigenous
people were overrepresented in Saskatchewan's suicide numbers, this
was an issue that affected everyone in the province.

For the next forty-four days, the group maintained a sacred fire and
welcomed visitors to the site. Two years earlier, the Justice for Our Stolen
Children Camp erected a tepee in the same spot. This was in response

to the acquittals of the people who had killed Colten Boushie and Tina Fontaine, but took on a wider call for justice within the notoriously damaging child welfare system, a system that has seen growing numbers of apprehensions in recent years. That camp stayed in Wascana Park from February to September, despite every effort from the province to have them leave. After arrests and forced dismantling of the tepee in June, the camp returned, now with six tepees and the support of a much wider community. The group was eventually forced out with a court order after 197 days.

Sitting with Tristen in the tepee as he drank the tea that kept him going through his fast, one had the sense of being with someone who was having a moment of purity. There were minor squabbles and complications at the camp, but his peaceful demeanour and focus on ceremony and the families of those who were lost kept people in good and generous spirits. Cabinet ministers Warren Kaeding and Lori Carr did come and meet with Tristen and try to convince him that Pillars for Life was sufficient.[23] The premier, however, refused to visit, even though the tepee was set up right across the parking lot from where he was working. Instead of listening to the tragic concerns brought forward, Moe's government took Tristen to court to try to get him and the tepee removed from Wascana Park. This time a judge ruled that this interfered with the constitutional right to protest and that Tristen could "complete his ceremonial fast and vigil without further incident."[24]

Before doing the walk, Tristen had started to feel fatalistic, as though there was nothing that could be done, that young people around him would just go on losing their lives to suicide. His experience with the walk changed his point of view. He saw promise in our increasing willingness to talk about mental health and self-care during the pandemic. And the response of so many people who encouraged him, who shared stories of their families or their own struggles with depression, gave him hope that people were ready to see a change. After forty-four days, the group held a ceremonial feast and dismantled the camp. The tepee was down, but the impression that Tristen, Chris, and the Walking With Our Angels group had left on Saskatchewan people was still standing.

The government would go on to vote in favour of Doyle's bill the third time we presented it in April 2021. We would discover later that they had not followed the law they had passed,[25] basically just slapping a strategy sticker on their pre-existing inadequate plan and calling it good enough. When this was revealed, they would then refuse to strike a public committee on mental health and suicide that would travel the province and hear from people what was needed in prevention and access to care.[26]

Healthy Minds, Healthy People

Why has the government shown so much resistance to doing this right? Why have they been willing to endure bad press and let a serious problem go unaddressed? It's hard to say, but I suspect it's because they understand the problem more than they let on. To truly address the suicide problem, you have to be willing to acknowledge the root causes of mental illness.

Reflecting on this brings me back to sitting at the Lighthouse recently with a man from a community in the far North. He'd come in to have a minor wound bandaged, and it would have been the easiest thing on a busy Friday morning to just patch him up and say, "See you next week." But something told me he wasn't doing so well and I dug a little deeper. He told me that a couple of days earlier, he'd nearly died by suicide and he was feeling really down. We sat and talked for nearly an hour and he told me his story. He spoke of being taken away from home by the RCMP to go to residential school, and about the trauma he carries from seeing one of his friends die right before him at school and being unable to do anything to help him. He told me of the physical attacks he'd been subjected to in his life and the serious mental and physical disabilities they caused. He told me of a life of poverty, how he was rejected by his home community, rejected by Saskatoon, rejected by pretty much everywhere but the Lighthouse and those few organizations that help people in the hardest situations. I spent that hour with him and I did what I could. We made a few calls and tried to get him some help. I tried to be that listening ear and tell him that whatever anybody says out there, in here we love you and we care about you. At the end of the session, I hoped I'd helped a bit, but I knew it was nowhere near what he needed. He'd experienced so much trauma and deprivation that couldn't be undone. We need to try to help people who have lived incredibly hard lives; we also need to make a lot of young lives easier.

As Tristen Durocher eloquently put it, "we have an undeniable right to a quality of life where we can make it to old age without having suicide, also known as hopelessness, be the leading cause of death."[27] Hopelessness – the sense that your life is worthless, that there is nothing to look forward to – is the experience of so many young people, and in particular young people in the North. To prevent suicide, we need to address the upstream factors that influence mental health, and that means being willing to investigate and address systemic inequities. We need to be honest about systemic racism and the intergenerational trauma of residential schools. The overrepresentation of Métis and First Nations people in poverty, in illness, in the penitential system: these are serious, long-standing, systemic problems. Tackling these inequities means confronting structures that benefit the people who currently enjoy wealth, power, and influence in our society.

Preventing suicide would also mean acknowledging the current lack of access to meaningful treatment for mental health and addictions. One of my greatest frustrations in family practice was hearing people say they were ready to quit drugs or alcohol, that they wanted to make a change, and telling them that was great, I might be able to get them into treatment in three to six months. When it came to getting people to see a psychiatrist, the waits were even longer. When someone is in the depths of a crisis and you say there's help coming months away, or that there are all kinds of hoops they need to jump through to be eligible, you might as well tell them their treatment is on Mars. We need to be able to get people help right away or we only return them to the substance use and despair they were finally willing to leave behind. One in five Canadians experiences mental illness each year. By the age of forty, half of all Canadians will experience at least one episode of mental illness.[28] On top of this tremendous human suffering, mental illness and addictions are estimated to cost Canada nearly $100 billion per year in added costs and decreased productivity.[29] Addressing the mental health crisis in Canada requires a willingness to understand what's driving the growth in hopelessness and a willingness to invest in making quality, evidence-based care accessible.

People's mental health has been profoundly impacted by COVID-19. It seems everyone's inner world has been rocked by changes in the outer. Loneliness, grief, fear, emotional conflict, and even the neurological effects of COVID itself[30] have added to the long-standing unaddressed burden of mental illness. Access that was awful before the pandemic became worse as clinics closed their doors and waiting lists soared. Patients can't get in to see their family doctor or a psychiatrist, can't afford counselling, and find themselves waiting among the heart attacks and broken legs in the emergency room. To respond to the growing mental health demands, we will need a major investment in prevention and primary care, psychological counselling, and crisis response, including expanded in-patient addictions care and dedicated emergency centres. The pandemic has exposed the fragility of our mental well-being. If we want a healthy future, we can't afford to leave our minds behind.

Eye of the Storm

Midway through the 2020 Saskatchewan provincial election, I found myself standing on stage shouting to the headlights of a parking lot full of honking cars.

Most people would describe me as a gentle, soft-spoken guy. That's an asset for a family doctor; it helps people to feel at ease, open up, and be vulnerable about things that are hard to discuss. To be a politician, I had to learn to turn up the volume a bit. That's a lot easier when it's a warm room. At party conventions and rallies, I can boom out the barn-burners, fired up by the infectious energy of excited supporters.

During the election, fear of other things infectious made those emotional moments harder to find. Hands were left unshaken, babies unkissed. Campaign launches and platform announcements were held in front of the legislature, in farmyards, parks, and parking lots. We held press conferences in places that tell a story, like a wheat field outside Regina where the former premier had promised to build an emergency care centre nearly ten years before, or outside a small-town school forced to close because a lack of adequate provincial precautions had left it vulnerable to a COVID outbreak. We then relied on traditional and social media to get that story to the people we couldn't meet in the usual way.

There was one moment, however, where that emotional high of connecting with a crowd happened in a way only a pandemic could provide. In the third week of the campaign, the campaign team set up a stage at a huge parking lot in Saskatoon, and another in Regina a few days later. Hundreds of people came out on chilly late October nights to be a part of the fun. Candidates in both cities acted as the emcees and there were musical acts to warm up the crowd, Ellen Froese and the Hot Toddies in Saskatoon, Megan Nash and the Best of Intentions in Regina.

At the Regina rally, former Alberta NDP premier Rachel Notley joined by video. After she spoke, I ran onto the stage. Like speaking in a theatre with the house lights down, I couldn't see anyone in the audience. Just darkness and the outlines of nearly 300 cars and trucks and semis in the crowd silhouetted in headlights. Clad in my parka on a freezing night, I gave one of the loudest speeches of my soft-spoken life. Applause lines became honk lines. I was so fired up I skipped over an entire page of my speech. No one noticed but me, of course. I ended by yelling, "Let's Put People First!" at the top of my lungs – the slogan and the volume both feeling perfectly natural despite the unnatural circumstances. Then, as Arthur White-Crummey reported in the *Regina Leader-Post*, Megan and the band came back onstage, finishing their set with a Fleetwood Mac song. They played "Dreams."[1]

We dreamed no little dreams, and I'm proud of the campaign we ran. We stayed positive, we had fun, and we proposed changes that would have made a real difference in Saskatchewan people's lives. The results wouldn't be what we'd hoped, but the dreams were good dreams.

The COVID Campaign

The trouble with a window of fine weather, it could be a lovely day or it could be the eye of the storm. Three days before the writ was dropped, Scott Moe tweeted: "Even though Justin Trudeau said Canada is now in the second wave of COVID-19, I remain confident we can avoid a significant second wave here in Saskatchewan if we all stay cautious and keep following good practices. What Saskatchewan people are doing has worked to date."[2] While this would prove to be tragically overconfident, no one knew that at the time. Saskatchewan had been spared the worst in the first wave. We were rightly proud of our collective response and relieved to have been spared the experiences of Ontario and Quebec, not to mention other countries that had been hit terribly hard.

As of the election call, we were six months into the pandemic and there had been a total of twenty-four recorded deaths from COVID in the province to date. Not a single death was recorded in the entire month of September. By election day that number was twenty-five, with a total of 2,800 confirmed cases. We would reach over ten times each of those numbers by the end of the second wave alone. At the time, however, we all shared in the naïveté and hope that maybe things would stay calm in Saskatchewan, and that our focus could shift to recovery. Over the summer, the Saskatchewan NDP had released a People-First Recovery plan looking at the policy choices that could help the economy rebound and people get back on their feet after a brutal spring.[3] This plan to invest in people as a stimulus for economic recovery was a stark contrast to the promised "austerity" from Finance Minister Donna Harpauer.[4]

Leading with People

The twenty-ninth Saskatchewan general election was officially called on September 29, 2020. Election day was set for October 26, as per the province's fixed election legislation. On the day the writ was dropped, I woke up early with energy to spare. I took a run around Wascana Lake, past where we would kick off the campaign in front of the legislature, and then back to my apartment to shower and suit up for the big launch. Out in front of the Queen Elizabeth II Gardens, I was joined by candidates from Regina to make our opening pitch. Looking back at photos, the six-foot spacing and cloth masks outdoors date the event quite clearly to summer 2020. There were no big surprises in that first speech, as we laid out our vision for health care, education, and the economy. The familiar refrains were met with familiar questions, as reporters asked me why we were bothering to position ourselves as a potential government. Why not just make the case that Saskatchewan needs a stronger opposition?

It was a fair question, but frustrating nonetheless. While we had hope of improving our seat count, winning a majority would require a miracle. The Sask Party had become a phenomenal political operation, dominating each of the last three provincial elections. The Saskatchewan NDP did not resemble the Orange Machine that had repeatedly put us in government since Tommy Douglas and the Co-operative Commonwealth

Federation (CCF) first formed a government in 1944. The Saskatchewan Party has been extremely successful at branding the NDP, the party of Medicare and public education, as a party that shuts hospitals and schools. It's a remarkably selective reading of history, one that ignores the state of bankruptcy the Grant Devine Progressive Conservatives handed to the Romanow government in the early 1990s, not to mention the stellar record of fiscal management of NDP governments. Regardless of the loose affiliation with the facts, many are convinced. There has also been a substantial and real rightward shift in the province's politics that, if not created by, was at least accelerated by the oil and potash booms of the 2010s.

Still, no matter how big the head start of your opponents, what could be less inspiring than saying to our team and our volunteers that we were running for second place? And what would it say to the people of the province to suggest they were so stuck in their ways we couldn't even imagine them changing their minds? No, even when the odds are long, you always run to win.

From that kickoff event, we headed off in the decal-wrapped cube van where the leader's tour team would spend most of the next month. Party supporters would later vote to name it the "Yes We Van." We stopped in Moose Jaw for another launch and some mainstreeting, went up to Saskatoon to put up the first lawn signs of the campaign, and then I headed home to put three-year-old Gus to bed. We kept up this kind of pace throughout the campaign, frequently hitting up four or more rural and urban campaigns a day. Each local campaign had a bubble, as did the central office, with people committing to see only their immediate family and their local team. Our "Bubble Buddy" crew consisted of Graham Reid behind the wheel (his safe driving would earn him the nickname Grandma Reid), chief of staff Adrienne King, press secretary Sally Housser, and photographer Josh Berson. It is a strange thing to spend a month driving around in a van with your face on the side and hours on end with a group you barely know, but thankfully these were delightful people and we had so much fun.

It was my first general election not only as leader but as a candidate as well. Still, I'd volunteered enough times to know things were different this time around. We would go out mainstreeting, but the streets were empty. At campaign stops, we'd meet a small group of volunteers outside because we couldn't invite everyone out to get fired up at a rally. At least we could safely go door to door, walking up the steps to knock and then backing up far enough that people would feel comfortable talking. People were keener to talk than ever, many saying no one had been to their door in forever and they were happy to just have someone listen. Still, so much that gets a team energized and could show momentum against a government was gone.

In the third week of the campaign, I stood surrounded by a group of people spaced out across the wooden medicine wheel at River Landing in Saskatoon. They had come to share their stories and join me in launching our full election platform. Kim was there, a teacher who saw her classrooms at a breaking point even before the pandemic. Sarah was there for her son, who had lost his educational assistant to budget cuts and was struggling with at-home learning. Lack of child care was forcing Lyndsay to choose between caring for her son or growing her business. Sharon was there, a First Nations senior and advocate concerned about the future for First Nations and Métis youth, while Abbas, a father of two, was alarmed at how everyday life was getting more expensive. Journeyman electrician Paul worried about jobs going to companies from outside Saskatchewan and wanted to see more opportunities in renewable energy.

I shared their stories, along with that of Cathy, a senior wondering how she'd be able to stay in her own home; Donna, who'd been waiting nearly three years for a hip replacement; and Sidney, who couldn't get an MRI because she didn't have the money to skip the line under the Sask Party's user-pay scheme. I spoke of nurses like Brenda, doing everything she could in a system failing her and her patients; of out-of-work construction workers in Moose Jaw; of people struggling with mental health and addictions in Regina; and of overwhelmed teachers in Prince Albert.

Our campaign slogan of "People First" was a recognition of whom we were there to serve and who needed our help. When I look back on the stories of the people who joined me that day, the social determinants of health leap out. Income, employment, education, housing, that's what people were talking to us about on the doorstep. So that's what we

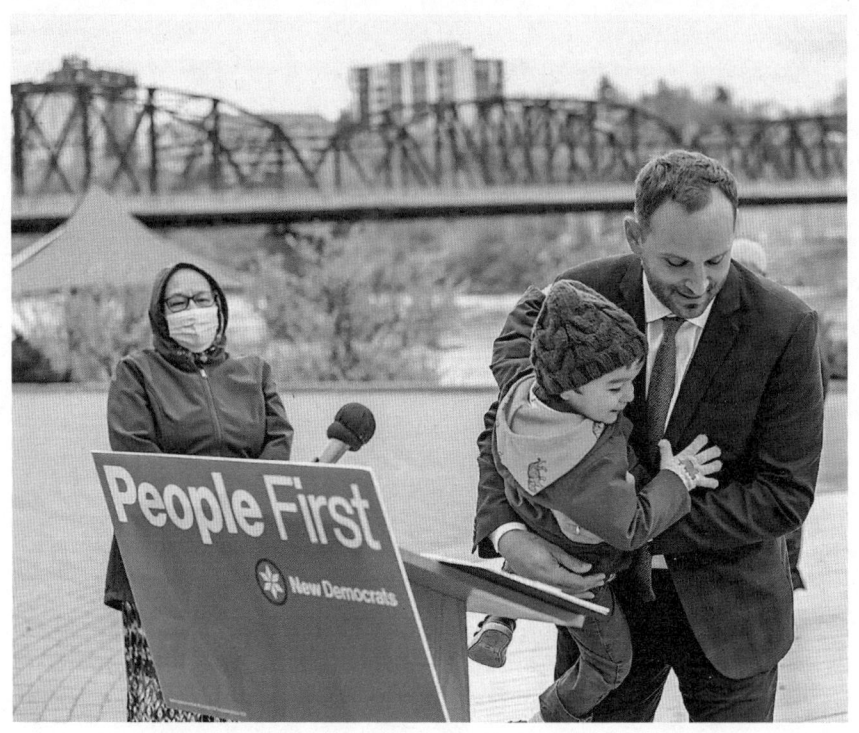

Gus joins the 2020 Saskatchewan NDP platform launch
(with Sharon Okeeweehow). October 2020 | *Joshua Berson*

put in the platform,[5] with commitments to increase the minimum wage, create jobs in renewable energy, fix our ailing health care system, expand home care, and get class sizes under control. It was a vision, built with the input of the community and party members, of the kind of place I want to live and raise my family. Speaking of whom, Mahli had brought Gus, who had just turned three, to watch the launch. Turns out he's not much of a spectator. Partway through my speech, he'd had enough and came running into my arms, just as I was talking about building a better life for Saskatchewan kids.

Competing Visions

With only two parties having seats in the Saskatchewan legislature, the provincial leaders' debate was a one-on-one showdown between me and

Scott Moe. The format consisted of a two-minute opening statement from each of us followed by questions on four topics to be chosen from COVID-19, the economy, health care, education, the environment, governance and leadership, and Indigenous issues. On each of these we would have forty-five seconds to respond, followed by three minutes of open debate. The open debate was the biggest concern, as I had no interest in another unwatchable performance of politicians shouting over each other.

For debate prep, the campaign brought in Jeff Ferrier, an experienced debate stand-in who had played Andrew Scheer for Jagmeet Singh and Andrew Wilkinson for John Horgan, to be our "Faux Moe." He was tough, sticking hard to Sask Party critiques of the NDP record and throwing me curveballs to knock me off my points. Between rounds of sparring, I worked with coaches Heather Fraser and Paul Degenstein of the NOW Group to find the best validating stories, pivot from what Moe wanted to talk about to our strong points, and deliver our main messages with confidence.

It was hard work to find the balance between being prepared enough to perform well but not so prepared as to be wooden and not genuine. This was helped by using Paul and Heather's CCS method: Connect, Contrast, Solve. You start by making an emotional link to the issue that makes it clear why it matters in the lives of real people, point out the flaws in your opponent's approach, and then make your pitch on how it could be done better. It's a deceptively simple approach they use in all their political communications, be they thirty-second ads, quick responses in scrums, or substantial speeches. Along with being a helpful way of organizing your thoughts when talking about complex and controversial questions, the emphasis on Connect reminds us that the audience we're trying to reach is made up of ordinary folks who are deciding how they should feel about the issue at hand. It's about speaking to people in a way that puts them and their values first.

The debate was held in the CBC studios in Wascana Park in Regina, with the legislature lit up and majestic in the background. The big open space made it natural to project a bit more, helping me overcome my soft-spoken Achilles heel. The other cure for that was singing. That's why before the big show, Mahli, Adrienne, Sally, and I spent the time in the green room dancing and belting out a few of our favourite tunes. This had become a routine on the campaign bus; before every press conference, we would sing "Dock of the Bay," which would put me in good voice and mood for the announcement and the subsequent scrum.

I said hello to each of the panelists and to the moderator, Molly Thomas from CTV's *W5*, then went and shook hands with Scott Moe. He was courteous and even friendly, and clearly at least as nervous as I was.

After opening statements, the first question of the night came from Adam Hunter of the CBC on whether we needed an indoor mask mandate. At the time cases were climbing quickly and the province had recently reduced the number of people allowed in private gatherings from thirty to fifteen. Moe said that the guidance for masking when you can't social distance was enough, while I expressed support for a mandate when necessary, calling for the thresholds for such a move to be laid out clearly. I then spoke of how strange it was that we were reducing gatherings to fifteen but sending kids into crowded classes of thirty, thirty-five, even forty kids and doing nothing to reduce those class sizes. After being cautioned by Molly that I was straying off the topic from COVID to schools, I made the case that this was indeed germane to COVID. I still laugh at that. I don't think I'd ever used the word "germane" in a sentence before and here I was trying to appeal to the regular guy using, as my mother likes to say, a nine-dollar word when a fifty-cent one would do.

First Nations University of Canada professor Merelda Fiddler-Potter asked us about the involvement of Indigenous people in the provincial economy. Here I referenced Australia's Closing the Gap[6] approach, where national, state, and territorial governments have committed to eliminating the inequality between Aboriginal and Torres Strait Islanders and the rest of the Australian population. It's a transparent, community-led model that could have a real impact in Saskatchewan and all of Canada. This led to perhaps the most heated moment of the debate, as I asked the premier why he voted against Doyle Vermette's suicide prevention bill and took Tristen Durocher to court instead of meeting with him. Even when pressed by Molly Thomas on whether he regretted that treatment, he said the visit from the ministers, who had essentially told Tristen to get off the legislature lawn, was good enough.

CTV journalist Alison Bamford asked about students who had slipped back several reading levels and teachers uncertain they'd be able to help them catch up by the end of the year. After Moe and I clashed about class sizes and the need for more teachers, the moderator asked the standard-issue question: How are you going to pay for it? Even when the need and the cost of failing to invest are clear, the assumption is that we can't afford nice things. As such, progressive parties are held to a different standard, with right-wing parties able to raise fears of "higher taxes," as Scott Moe did with a smirk, even when his own party had increased the provincial sales tax only a couple of years earlier. Some of this framing is so baked in that it's extremely challenging to shift the discussion to the return on social investment without the assumption, contrary to the historical record, that parties on the left simply run up deficits.

The final set of questions was on the overdose crisis. At that point in 2020, over twice as many people had died in Saskatchewan from overdoses than from COVID, car accidents, and impaired driving combined. I spoke of families who had lost sons and daughters, and how, as a parent, you do everything you can to set kids on a good path, but the fear is always there. Harm reduction, a crystal meth and opioid strategy, and the establishment of dedicated mental health and addictions emergency rooms are desperately needed. The debate then turned to safe consumption sites, something the province has. I quoted Marie Agioritis, Saskatchewan vice-chair of Moms Stop the Harm[7] and mother of a young man who had died from an overdose, who told me, "You can't help people get off drugs if they're dead." By preventing overdose and infections like HIV and hepatitis C, safe consumption sites can be an important tool in keeping people alive and connecting them to the supports they need to get clean.

In closing statements, Moe contrasted his plans with his version of the NDP record from the 1990s. I invited people to be part of a needed change, to build a better future together. While there were no stop-the-presses knockout punches, the debate felt great. There were a couple of hot moments, but it never degenerated into the kind of off-putting, incoherent shouting match I'd feared it could. I'd been able to present a clear vision and put the premier on his heels with some tough direct questions, and to come across as confident and professional. The campaign team was over the moon, thrilled with how well it had gone.

The euphoria wouldn't last. The next day's headline wasn't a positive review, or even a "leaders clash in provincial debate." Instead, the *Regina Leader-Post* front-page story was a poll commissioned by its parent company, Postmedia, indicating that the Sask Party was set to win the election with a massive majority. I have no idea how these editorial decisions are made, but it was hard not to see a thumb on the scale. The debate is the one moment an opposition party has a chance to make a splash and give people the impression they do have a choice. This polling story was perfectly timed to throw cold water on any such momentum.

As discouraging as that was, our team powered through, focused on election day. Even if the coverage wasn't what we'd hoped, the response on the doorstep changed. The debate had made an impression. Later that week, Mahli and I voted in the advance polls. We walked the three blocks from my Saskatoon campaign office to the polling station with camera operators and photographers running alongside us. The last few days of the campaign were a blur of whistle stops and outdoor visits with candidates and supporters in the parking lots of urban campaign headquarters, in a farmyard in Southey at sundown, and after dark in downtown North Battleford.

On election day we knocked on doors, trying to encourage those who hadn't mailed in their ballot or made it out to advanced polls to get out and vote. I met a few people who couldn't vote because they were in isolation as COVID contacts or had caught the virus themselves. It's hard to know which communities and voters were less likely to make it out to vote, but turnout dropped by 5 percent from the previous provincial election.

In the afternoon I joined the team at a Saskatoon hotel. I sat with Adrienne King and provincial campaign manager Trevor McKenzie-Smith, looking at polling that showed us winning between fifteen and twenty seats and daydreaming about what that could mean. It was a far cry from government, but it would have meant more MLAs and more staff to do the work, a chance to be a truly effective opposition and a sense we were building to something more.

Upstairs in the hotel, I ironed my shirt while watching the early results come in with Abe and Mahli. Things started out well, with us leading in seventeen or eighteen seats for a while, not as high as we'd hoped, but progress. As the night wore on, it got worse. We dropped to twelve seats by early evening, and I went down to the hotel conference room to give my concession speech.

The Hope That'll Kill You

Unlike other elections, there wasn't a throng of supporters and candidates there to cheer for our efforts. There was no "victory party," just a room full of television cameras and reporters. Mahli joined me at the podium, and I did my best to encourage people, to remind the 30 percent of the population that did support us, that did vote for change, that their vote counts. But I couldn't hide my disappointment.

When I went to bed on election night, I was leading in my seat of Saskatoon Meewasin. When I woke up, I was behind by eighty-three votes. We were fairly confident that, with many mail-in votes yet to be counted, we would ultimately hold the seat. Still, it was a harsh wake-up call to the fact that, despite the efforts of so many, the battle ahead would be longer and tougher, with no more resources than we had going in.

Politicians are the worst assessors of the outcomes of contests they were a part of, but for what it's worth, here's my mine. We'd run a campaign with no major blunders and a positive message, but the truth is, it was never there for us. The middle of a crisis is a challenging time to sell a message of change. COVID and our recovery from it were the biggest issues, and while that would change drastically in the following year, in the fall of 2020 Saskatchewan was a success story. There was also a significant "rally 'round the flag" effect, with incumbent governments returning with larger majorities in places like New Brunswick and British Columbia, and in national elections in New Zealand. The one major exception, despite his delusions to the contrary, was then US president Donald Trump, whose disastrous handling of the pandemic contributed to his loss. Holding our ground, while no one's idea of success, was likely all we could hope for.

When the final results were returned in the 2020 Saskatchewan provincial election, holding our ground is what happened. We won thirteen seats and 31 percent of the vote. That compares with the two previous elections that had seen the Saskatchewan NDP win nine seats and 32 percent of the vote under Dwain Lingenfelter in 2011, and ten seats and 30 percent of the vote under Cam Broten in 2016. Both of those leaders had lost their seats, triggering leadership races. That meant we'd earned more votes and seats than in the previous election and held the leader's seat for the first time in a decade. However, since we'd added three seats in by-elections since 2016, there were no gains from before the writ was dropped.

Ultimately, it's the hope that kills you. The polling had us believing we would see more growth. Failing to meet those expectations left the party dispirited and demoralized. The disappointing results set the stage for some within the party to campaign actively against my continuing in my role. This couldn't have come at a worse time, turning us inward at the very moment the province would go from among the best pandemic response in the country to the very worst. Given the urgent need to be an effective opposition in the face of a rising second wave, dispirited and demoralized was the last thing we needed to be.

My point is not to bright-side or to relitigate the election here. There is no court of appeal on the people's decision. Whether our campaign or plan was better, our results were worse. We lost. But it's worth remembering that the outcome of the election does not invalidate the debate leading up to it. People have a binary choice at the ballot box: if they like a quarter of one party's platform and three-quarters of the other, they don't get to divide their vote to reflect those sympathies. And in the two-party system that has emerged in Saskatchewan, any nuance in public desire is eliminated in the all-or-nothing distribution of legislative power. My point in reviewing the election campaign is that the issues we talked about then are still worth talking about today. Ideas like paid sick leave, expanded home care, or the "Renew Saskatchewan" home renewable energy plan were worth proposing then and are still worth pursuing today. Simply because they didn't carry the day in our elections as structured doesn't mean they should be discarded and forgotten. When it comes to COVID, I can't help but wonder what might have been for the province had the outcome on election day been different. I remain confident an NDP government would have handled the pandemic far better, but this is not a story of what might have been; it's the story of what was.

In the days leading up to the election, COVID numbers were rising quickly. Despite a record number of new cases the day before, Scott Moe promised at his final campaign stop in Regina that there would be no more shutdowns.[8] In his acceptance speech on election night, he didn't address the 30 percent of Saskatchewan people who had voted for the official opposition and promise he would hear them out. Instead, he spoke to the 3 percent who had voted for the far-right separatist Buffalo Party, saying that "we share your frustrations, and we share many of your objectives."[9] This signalled the further shift to the right that he would take in the years to follow. It also set the stage for the inaction that would characterize the coming waves. The eye of the storm had passed, the wind was blowing wildly, and the big waves were about to come crashing down.

Second Wave

OCTOBER 2020 – JANUARY 2021

I have no idea what's awaiting me,
or what will happen when this all ends.
For the moment I know this: there are
sick people and they need curing.

– Albert Camus, *The Plague*

Total cases in Canada	588,935
Total cases in Saskatchewan	10,584
Deaths from COVID in Canada	10,494
Deaths from COVID in Saskatchewan	280

Provincial Public Health Measures

October 13, 2020	Private gatherings limited to fifteen people
November 6, 2020	Mask mandate introduced in Saskatoon, Prince Albert, and Regina
November 19, 2020	Mask mandate expanded province-wide
	Private gathering limits reduced to five
	Visitation to long-term care homes suspended
November 25, 2020	Restaurants and bars limited to four people per table
	Performance venues, indoor public events, places of worship limited to thirty people
	Competitions, recitals, etc. suspended; practice and training permitted in groups of eight or less
December 3, 2020	SHA escalates surge response
December 17, 2020	Inter-household gatherings prohibited
December 25, 2020	Retail services limited to 50 percent capacity, large retail to 25 percent

Ignoring the Signs

On November 24, 2020, Neil Sasakamoose posted a video to Facebook. Choking back tears, he told the province that his father was gone. Fred Sasakamoose was a Saskatchewan legend, the first Treaty Indian to play in the National Hockey League. Despite playing only a handful of games for the Chicago Blackhawks, he was a trailblazer, a beacon to generations of young players both through his own career and through his work establishing hockey opportunities for First Nations youth.

Fred stayed true to his roots, returning to his home community of Ahtahkakoop Cree Nation and raising nine children with his wife, Loretta. He served on band council and as Chief, and openly shared his experiences of abuse at St. Michael's Residential School with the Truth and Reconciliation Commission.

I spoke with Neil a couple of months after his father's death. He described a complex relationship with a towering figure, larger than life, and deep frustration over an avoidable, preventable loss. But mostly he felt for his dad. "My dad suffered," he said, taking a long pause to fight back the tears. "He suffered."

A funeral on reserve had brought the virus into the community. Neil's nephew, who lived with his grandparents, got sick a few days later, with a high fever and a severe enough headache that he called an ambulance. His symptoms were dismissed as not serious and the ambulance left. The next day, Fred started to feel sick at church. The nephew got tested that Wednesday, a test that turned out to be positive, but in a failure that highlights the lack of organization and capacity in testing at the time, eighty-five- and eighty-six-year-old Loretta and Fred weren't tested, even though Fred was already sick.

As the week went on, Fred's symptoms got worse. Neil phoned home to his dad, who answered, "He...ll...o...my...boy." That's when Neil knew something was really wrong. His dad was always moving, always busy. Even in the days before he went into hospital, he'd been out clearing snow and splitting firewood. Now here he was lying flat, hardly able to push out a single word. Neil broke the news to him that he had COVID-19 and needed to get to the hospital. This was on a Friday, and over the weekend, his breathing worsened and his oxygen saturation levels continued to fall.

Monday morning Fred had a phone call with Elders and with his brothers Peter, who lives in Kamloops, British Columbia, and Leo from Edmonton. Neil described how close Fred was with his brothers as "small-kid close, residential-school-survivor close." On that call, they prayed, and Fred vowed to beat the illness. But this was one opponent too strong even for the determination of the man they called Chief Thunderstick.

That Tuesday morning at 6 a.m., Neil got a call from the hospital. He learned that Fred was doing very badly. He was told that if they didn't insert a tube to breathe for him, he would die, and even if they did, the chances of recovery were extremely low. Neil talked to his dad on the phone and told him he loved him. He'd never said that before, even though they were close. They just didn't talk that way, but he wanted Fred to know. He asked Fred what he wanted to do. Fred was afraid to die, but he knew his time had come. "You know what," he said, "I'm ready to go. I want to go to heaven now."

That afternoon, Fred's nurse was checking on him. He asked her to get him some water and when she came back, he was gone.

Fred's loss was felt far and wide. An article in the *New York Times* recounted his outsized impact on the lives of First Nations people and on the world of hockey.[1] After so much struggle, having risen above the hardships to excel in his sport, to raise nine children and 128 grand-children and great-grandchildren, to become a leader in his community,

Fred had left his mark. In April 2021, his book *Call Me Indian*[2] was released and became a national bestseller, keeping his story alive, but sadly without him here to see its success and know how his legacy lives on.

Neil found some peace in knowing his father was ready to go. It wasn't always easy to be Fred's son – there were hard years of alcoholism and anger – but Neil has found clarity and been able to forgive him. He wants to make sure Fred isn't forgotten. He threw himself into supporting vaccination efforts, establishing a partnership between the Battlefords Agency Tribal Chiefs, the Prince Albert Grand Council, and the Saskatoon Tribal Council to run vaccine clinics and promote vaccination in First Nations communities.[3] Alongside this positive outlet, anger and frustration remained at what happened to his father.

Neil knew that if Fred had been tested earlier, if he'd gotten treatment sooner, he might still be with us. If the community had been better protected from the spread of COVID-19 in the first place, he might still be with us. He wanted answers on how this happened, and he's not the only one. Families across Saskatchewan are mourning the loss of a loved one or dealing with ongoing health problems from COVID-19. These families deserve to know what decisions were made and why, to have a full understanding of the choices made that led to things going as badly as they did.

On the Horizon

Modelling from the SHA in October and November had predicted an out-of-control second wave in Saskatchewan. That modelling wasn't shared with physicians or the public, nor did it lead the government to take the action needed to prevent that outcome. When *Regina Leader-Post* reporter Arthur White-Crummey's freedom of information request uncovered this, Health Minister Paul Merriman said: "At the time, we wanted to make sure that we were reacting to what we saw, not what could come on the horizon."[4] It's hard to imagine a statement more revealing of the government's approach, or more out of line with the principles of public health and prevention. Public health is all about the horizon. It's about getting ahead of a problem before it becomes one.

By the time you can "see" something, by the time there is evidence of widespread illness from an infectious disease, the game is already lost.

The modelling in question was from October 29, three days after the provincial election. We don't know what modelling was being done prior to the election. It's possible it was being done and seen by the premier; it's possible that work had been paused for the election. Neither possibility would be particularly impressive. Nonetheless, the post-election projections showed a sharp spike in cases, hospitalizations, and deaths in the coming weeks. Case counts of 120 or 200 may seem small post-Omicron, but at the time we were used to single-digit daily cases, and with vaccines and treatment still unavailable, this represented a significant risk. Regular updates of these projections were provided to the SHA and government, but nothing was shared with the public until a press conference three weeks later, on November 19.[5] At that time, the public presentation included an "optimistic scenario" that hadn't been included in a similar presentation to doctors and was already two weeks out of date.[6]

In the meantime, the province slowly began to respond to the growing reality of a second wave. On November 6, a mask mandate was introduced for Regina, Saskatoon, and Prince Albert; this was expanded to the entire province on November 19. Masking in schools, and gathering limits in homes, restaurants, places of worship, and other public venues were introduced on November 25. Inter-household gatherings would be prohibited on December 17 and retail store capacity limited as of Christmas Day. This slow trickling of new interventions tracked a steadily climbing rate of community transmission of the virus, hospitalizations, and deaths. Prior to the provincial election, twenty-five people had died from COVID in the province; over ten times that many were lost by the end of January. Testing and tracing, having been reduced in capacity over the summer rather than strengthened in preparation for the fall, were unable to keep up with demand. Outbreaks in schools, long-term care centres, and prisons were daily occurrences. Restrictions had to continue for months instead of being brought in quickly and effectively before things got out of control. We had ignored the signs on the horizon and were stuck reacting to what we saw, and what we saw was ugly.

Circuit Breaker

It didn't have to be that way. There was a different path available, and the voices calling for it were loud, clear, and credible. Drawing on models being used elsewhere and advice from public health experts in the province, in mid-November I called for a three-week "circuit breaker," a short-term set of restrictions that included closure of non-essential businesses, reduction of capacity in essential businesses, reduction of class sizes, and supports for businesses to maintain payroll and for workers who were off work.[7] This was designed to quickly and effectively reduce transmission and timed to try to avoid having the worst of times over the Christmas holidays. Not surprisingly, the government wasn't interested in hearing this from me as opposition leader, but it was not only political voices calling for action.

Just days earlier, a group of doctors had written a letter that would be signed by over 400 of their colleagues across the province.[8] I reproduce that letter here in full as it shows that another path was being clearly presented, and highlights the role of health care professionals as advocates throughout the pandemic.

Dear Premier Moe, Minister Merriman, and Dr. Shahab,

Re: A call for leadership to combat the rapid spread of COVID-19 in Saskatchewan

In the past 30 days, the number of active COVID-19 cases in Saskatchewan has increased 700% to 1,289. Our hospitals are full, in part due to a 517% increase in COVID-19 admissions. Saskatoon ICUs are at 130% capacity and are diverting patients. It is becoming increasingly clear to us, physicians from across Saskatchewan, that we are losing the battle against this virus. If more is not done to change our course we are confident that winter will bring overflowing hospitals, canceled surgeries, overwhelmed health care providers, and needless deaths.

We appreciate that, in battling this epidemic, there are no easy solutions. From the inconvenience of wearing masks, to the isolation of social distancing and quarantine, to the harms felt by local businesses with every escalation in restrictions, we know that doing more will be difficult for Saskatchewan people. However, the lives of our friends and neighbours are on the line.

As our newly re-elected government, we look to you for leadership. Models of successful interventions that could be applied in Saskatchewan are available from Atlantic Canada, New Zealand, Australia, South Korea, and more. We know that you have the expertise needed to apply them. A common thread in each successful region and country is the clear and consistent leadership and communication of an empathetic government guided by a solid foundation of science and expert medical opinion.

Both action and inaction will be criticized. We humbly ask you to act with sufficient force to reverse the rising daily case counts while also detailing how and when we would escalate our interventions even further. Making decisions, even when difficult, is the hallmark of strong leadership. The lives and livelihoods of Saskatchewan people depend upon you.

Sincerely, 402 Saskatchewan Physicians[9]

A few days later, having seen only the minor changes of broadened mask mandates and an earlier last call for alcohol sales in bars,[10] the group called for specific measures to enhance testing and tracing and to close businesses that posed a high risk for transmission.[11] This too was signed by over 400 doctors and, though dismissed by the government as not representing the views of all physicians, aligned with a position paper written by the president of the Saskatchewan Medical Association and endorsed by the College of Physicians and Surgeons of Saskatchewan, College of Family Physicians of Canada (Saskatchewan Chapter), Saskatchewan Registered Nurses' Association, Saskatchewan Union of Nurses, Pharmacy Association of Saskatchewan, and Saskatchewan College of Pharmacy Professionals.[12]

This was just one example of many collective and individual efforts by doctors, nurses, and others in the health professions to speak out for wise action in the face of COVID-19. Earlier, another group of docs had reached out to Saskatchewan businesses, urging them to employ practices that would keep their customers and staff safe.[13] And in 2021, physicians in leadership positions, including the province's medical officers of health, would become much more vocal in stating their frustrations and giving direction for a better response to the fourth wave.

A leader among these public physician voices was Dr. Hassan Masri, an intensive care specialist in Saskatoon. He started posting myth-buster videos in March 2020,[14] gathering a large following for his frank and funny straight talk on COVID. He later became one of the faces of the province's "Stick It to COVID" campaign before his frustration with the mishandling of the fourth wave led him to be more overtly critical of the Saskatchewan Party. He eventually chose to leave Saskatchewan for Ontario in 2022, directly citing Scott Moe's "failed leadership" during the pandemic as one of the driving factors.[15]

Dr. Masri, epidemiologists Cory Neudorf and Nazeem Muhajarine, family doctor Carla Holinaty, public health nurse Carolyn Brost Strom, ER docs Brent Thoma and Paul Olszynski, child psychiatrist Tamara Hinz – these are just a few of the many who put their professional reputations on the line and faced pushback online for speaking out about the challenges facing health care and the risks to public health. Frequently health professionals stay out of the fray of political debates, wanting to maintain their neutrality and objectivity. There may also be fear of retaliation from governments that aren't receptive to criticism. The urgency of the pandemic made it impossible to keep that silence. It will be interesting to see what impact that will have on the culture of the health professions and continued advocacy in the future. Given the rise of misinformation and the ability of those promoting false narratives on health care to gain large audiences and, in the case of Alberta premier Danielle Smith, high elected office, that evidence-based advocacy will be more important than ever.

For those who might suggest this is a departure from their professional roles, it's worth noting that being a health advocate is considered central to the role of physician. The Royal College of Physicians and Surgeons of Canada description of the health advocate role points out that "physicians are accountable to society and recognize their duty to contribute to efforts to improve the health and well-being of their patients, their communities, and the broader populations they serve."[16] Despite being a recognized core competency, this recent advocacy on the part of health care providers is unlike anything I'd seen in my career. And it happened all across the country, with examples like Protect Our Province Alberta giving COVID briefings when Alberta had stopped doing so in the summer of 2021,[17] or the modelling and advocacy of Dr. Jennifer Kwan in Ontario and her work with Doctors for Justice in Long-Term Care.[18] At one point in the fourth wave, Scott Moe suggested that the medical community should focus their advocacy on providing COVID-19 information to the public rather than challenging the government's approach. This struck a particularly sour note with those advocates and frontline providers who had been spending so much time sharing that information while also dealing with the fallout of COVID-19 in health care. Saskatchewan Union of Nurses president Tracy Zambory called the comments "tone deaf," and "a real blow to an already exhausted, tired workforce that has been showing up consistently since March 2020."[19]

The highest-profile physician voices have been those of chief medical health officers (CMHOs) across the country. Some of these voices, such as Dr. Bonnie Henry in British Columbia, have been more independent, able to make decisions or announcements on their own. Others, including Saskatchewan's Dr. Saqib Shahab, have been more at the mercy of their employers. This is not only a matter of perception but a function of different legislation in the different provinces. A 2018 paper in the *Canadian Journal of Public Health* described three categories of chief medical health officer: the "Loyal Executive," whose function consists of advising the minister of health and designing the province's public health response; "Everyone's Expert," who advises as well but also has a role of direct, independent communication with the public and the legislature on matters of public health; and the "Technical Officer."[20] This final model has neither the official advisory role nor the authority to communicate directly to the legislature or the public. It is in this final category that the Saskatchewan *Public Health Act* places Dr. Shahab. While he was frequently put in the position of advising and of communicating with the public, these were "at pleasure" functions, entirely dependent on the will of the premier or the minister of health. He may have been the face of the decisions, but the final call on what to do and what to say came down to his employers. *Regina Leader-Post* columnist Sarath Peiris penned an op-ed during the fourth wave that outlined these concerns well. In response to the absence of the chief medical health officer from the public eye for several weeks, and the fact that Saskatchewan's policies were clearly out of step with expert opinion, he wrote of Dr. Shahab that "it was clear that his role was as a government employee, not as an independent watchdog of the public interest."[21]

As much as he didn't have the independence or authority to make or communicate the public health decisions himself, Dr. Shahab had to wear them, taking the heat when those choices were not well received. This included criticism from those who felt the government was not doing enough, and more viciously from those who thought too much was being done. A so-called freedom rally outside the Saskatchewan legislature in December 2020 featured someone yelling racist comments about Dr. Shahab, mocking the pronunciation of his name, and referring to him disparagingly as a foreigner.[22]

A few weeks later that ugliness turned into something more menacing as protesters picketed outside Dr. Shahab's home. To his credit, Premier Moe was fierce in his defence of Dr. Shahab and his criticism of these protesters, rightly describing them as "a group of idiots."[23] That same group was outside the legislature most days for months, blaring music, holding signs accusing those delivering vaccines of murder, and shouting at MLAs as we went to our cars. They were idiots there as well, but that's the place for protest, that's the public square. It's not at someone's home and it's not outside hospitals, as they would do in later months. This was a particularly repulsive development, where people going in to see their loved ones sick in the ICU or coming home from a twelve-hour shift caring for the sick had to run the gauntlet of placards saying that COVID wasn't real. For that reason, we called for legislation that would bar protests outside of hospitals, legislation that the government would agree to a couple of months later.[24]

Returning to Dr. Shahab's situation, it was extremely disturbing to see him, an unelected provincial employee, personally harassed for doing his job. It was also encouraging to see the way that Saskatchewan people stood up for him. People across the province spoke out against the actions of these protesters and in praise of the work he had done. The local Tim Hortons even made a sweater-vest donut in his honour.[25]

As admirable as it is for the premier and others to have Dr. Shahab's back when he faces blowback, there is a larger question here. Why is a non-elected public servant without the independence to make decisions or communicate to the public without government oversight taking this kind of heat? We have a situation where politicians can hide behind public health officials for cover from unpopular decisions, point the finger at them if things don't go well, take credit for popular choices or for good results, and ignore the officials when doing the right thing for health is not seen to be in their political interest. We must make a choice: Do we want our public health leadership to simply give advice and let the politicians decide, or do we want them to lead? If it's only advice, then it should be the politicians who take responsibility, and the health officers can stay out of the public conversation. Or we can give CMHOs more independence and the freedom to share their advice publicly and the politicians are then judged on whether they follow that advice rather than allowing them to shape it behind the scenes. Right now, with rec-ommendations made behind closed doors and the CMHOs having to carry the political message to the public, we have the worst of both worlds: public health experts being held accountable for decisions they don't have the power to make. As Peiris proposed, "it's time to designate chief health officers as independent officers of the legislature, serving a watchdog role comparable to that of provincial auditors, with their re-ports being made public documents."[26] Concerns about independence and interference emerged again in April 2023, when Saskatchewan's minister of rural and remote health announced in a scrum that masking requirements were removed from hospitals. Columnist Murray Mandryk wrote in response that "we need to be sure such recommendations are independently made and not somehow driven by politicians trying to score points for lifting masking restrictions."[27]

On the Ward Again

As others were answering the call to add advocacy to their full-time clinical vocations, I was adding clinical service back into my advocacy. In November 2020 an urgent email was sent to all SHA physicians from the pandemic leadership saying, "We need your help! As COVID-19 numbers increase in the hospital, clinical service delivery needs are growing. We need your help in the areas of Hospital, Field Hospital, Emergency and ICU." I signed up and did three days of training on the respirology service at Royal University Hospital (RUH) and the internal medicine and COVID ward services at St. Paul's Hospital. I would later join a team of what are called "house officers" at RUH. This service was added during the pandemic to provide backup to the overtaxed internal medicine teams.

The training and my first shifts were like going back in time and becoming a resident or medical student again. I followed the attending physicians around on rounds, trying to be useful but mostly just asking dumb questions. Some of the patients and staff recognized me and wanted to talk politics, but most just saw another mask and a set of scrubs. On shift, I would round on patients, making sure I knew the back story of everyone on the unit in case I got called during the night. Not all the patients on our service had COVID, but several did. Many were long-term care patients waiting for placement, others were HIV-positive and on prolonged antibiotics for endocarditis or osteomyelitis. Once I'd read all the charts and chatted with the nurses, I'd retire to the call room on the fourth floor of the old hospital. When I was training and in practice, that was the obstetrics wing, and memories of the many long nights and hundreds of deliveries there came flooding back as I ate my cafeteria supper in the little overnight call room. The fact that I'd get a kick out of doing "real doctor" things like ordering meds and labs and examining patients reminded me how long it had been since I'd practised at any level of intensity. I was very grateful for the medical and nursing staff who could have treated me like a dilettante or a tourist. Instead, they fully welcomed me on the team and seemed to genuinely appreciate the physician voice in the public sphere and the willingness to lend a hand on the frontlines, however limited that contribution might be.

Case Conference

I met Dr. Monga Palangi on my first shift on the COVID-19 ward in the fifth-floor observation unit of RUH. Observation units are for patients

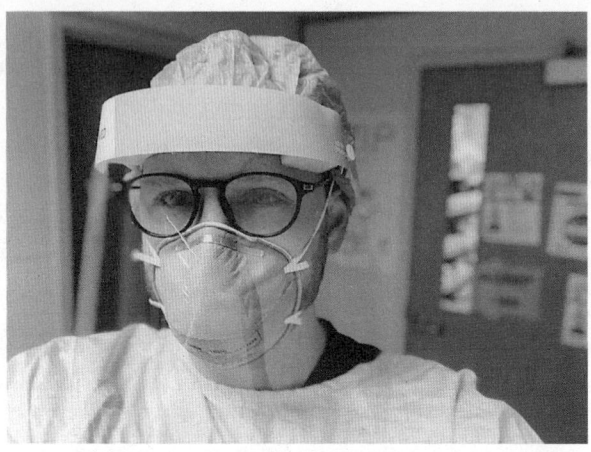

**Donning PPE to enter the COVID observation ward,
Royal University Hospital. February 2021**

who are too sick to be in the regular ward, but not quite sick enough for intensive care. This particular unit is for COVID-19 patients whose treatment includes certain kinds of high-flow oxygen therapy. For a patient struggling to breathe, a concentrated stream of oxygen can be life-saving. It is also what we call an "aerosol generating medical procedure" because the turbulent airflow sends the SARS-CoV-2 virus that causes COVID-19 disease flying throughout the room. As you can imagine, the infection control precautions in those units are very strict.

It was my first shift on the COVID ward in response to calls from the Saskatchewan Health Authority for doctors to assist. The entrance to the observation unit – located in what was the newborn nursery back when I was a medical trainee at the same hospital – is in a back hallway on the fifth floor. Just outside, there is a long table laden with PPE. Face shields, hair covers, latex gloves, bright yellow gowns, and various kinds of N95 masks are laid out in boxes. As I prepared to go in, my mind went back to the "donning and doffing" videos everyone working with patients has studied carefully. They show you how to carefully put things on in the right order, using hand sanitizer at every step to be sure you are fully protected. Getting this right protects you from getting infected, avoids bringing the virus into a patient's room, or in the case of this unit, bringing it out to the rest of the hospital and infecting other patients and staff.

Dr. Palangi is a family physician, originally from the Democratic Republic of the Congo. He trained in medicine there, moved to South Africa, where he studied family medicine and practised for twenty years, and then came to Saskatchewan in 2010. He first worked in the town of Leader, and since August 2020 has been practising in the west central community of Kindersley. Like all Saskatchewan doctors, his practice changed dramatically in 2020. He adapted to seeing patients virtually when possible and protecting himself in new ways when doing physical exams or treating patients in hospital.

Training and practising in Congo in the 1970s and '80s, and later in South Africa, this was not his first pandemic. He had seen the rise of HIV and how he and his fellow health care workers had to change their practices to protect themselves. He saw the parallels with today's situation, with the initial doubts and suspicion followed by people being forced to take the illness seriously as it became widespread. I recall working in a rural hospital in Mozambique before antiretrovirals were widely available, watching patients wither and die from AIDS without anything to offer them but comfort measures. Despite the seriousness of the illness, it was extremely challenging to convince people to change their normal patterns of behaviour, even when their friends and family were becoming ill.

I would discuss these pandemic parallels with Dr. Palangi later, but that's not what we were talking about that day. It's not uncommon to meet up with a colleague on the ward to discuss patient care. That's not how or why I met Dr. Palangi. He wasn't there working to assist patients, he was simply working hard to breathe, lying on his face in the prone position that had been discovered to help patients with COVID-19 pneumonia improve their oxygen saturation. I sat beside his bed to see how he was doing, to see if there was anything he needed. I also asked him about his story, curious how a family physician came to be hospitalized with COVID-19. He told me, between laboured breaths, that he'd been very careful, isolating at home with family and exercising caution at work, but that he was quite certain he'd caught the virus while treating patients as a family doctor in Kindersley.

A few weeks later, after he'd been discharged home from hospital, I spoke with Dr. Palangi and his wife, Sherstin, by phone. He was calm and measured in his description of his experience, but there were moments in the recounting of his story that betrayed profound emotion and displayed the fatigue and confusion that he is struggling to move past. He had lost forty or fifty pounds in hospital, the fight for each and every breath wearing down his muscles. He'd gone from looking too young for his sixty-six years to describing himself as having aged ten years.

He believes it was in the Kindersley hospital that he contracted the SARS-CoV-2 virus. There was an outbreak in the Kindersley area and three patients became positive in hospital. Dr. Palangi was doing telephone appointments in a shared space with other physician colleagues, and they removed their masks to do this work. One of the other doctors tested positive on January 22 and Dr. Palangi was identified as a close contact and told to isolate for fourteen days.

That Monday, Monga tried to do a telephone clinic but had to stop as he felt sick and weak. He had a fever of thirty-nine degrees, terrible chills, muscle aches, and fatigue. He would lie on the couch covered with a blanket, unable to get warm. He stayed home and tried to recover, and even thought he might be getting better as the fever broke, but on February 3, he started to have difficulty breathing. He went to the Kindersley hospital, where they told him his oxygen saturation was too low and that if they didn't send him to Saskatoon, he might not make it. While there are many ways that COVID-19 can make someone very sick, respiratory failure is the most common danger as the virus inflames the lungs so much that they can't deliver oxygen into the bloodstream. The average person's oxygen saturation percentage is in the high nineties. Monga's was dropping into the seventies.

He stayed for two weeks in RUH, first in a regular ward room and later in the observation unit. He described how frightening it was to be in that unit, particularly as a doctor. A curtain separated him from the other patients, but he could hear the codes being called overhead, and hear the medical team shouting instructions and knew exactly what they meant. He would hear the code called, hear all the activity, then silence as the bed was pushed away. He referred to it as being in a "death room," and how his mortality was more present than he'd ever imagined. Doctors, being in the position of caring for everyone else's health, often carry with them a sense of invincibility, as though sickness is something that happens to their patients, not to them. This natural psychological protection was torn away from Dr. Palangi in his hospital bed. There were moments where he felt ready to give up entirely, thinking that dying was inevitable and he was just too tired to keep fighting.

Fortunately, he never gave up, and after two weeks he didn't need as much oxygen support and was transferred back to Kindersley hospital. When we spoke in March 2021, he was just starting to settle into life back at home. His wife is an RN and she and their two children, aged two and four, had also contracted COVID-19. They'd recovered quickly and were now adjusting to Monga's ongoing illness. He was still short of breath and requiring oxygen at times, but his endurance and memory were slowly improving. He was just starting to think about going back to work, but with some trepidation. He still didn't feel as sharp as usual, and he also knew that going back to work would not be easy. Like so many rural practices, his was extremely busy and challenging and constantly understaffed. A group that should include seven doctors had only three, and he attributes some of the severity of his illness to the burnout he was experiencing before he got sick.

Hearing Dr. Palangi's story brought me back to the first days of the pandemic in Saskatchewan and the very legitimate fears of health care workers as we watched what was happening around the world. Over 150 Italian physicians, many of them general practitioners assisting with the response, died in the first weeks of the outbreaks there. Health systems around the world were being overwhelmed. People on the frontlines were put in the impossible position of deciding whether each specific patient should be put on a scarce ventilator or whether it should be saved for someone more likely to recover.

We're incredibly grateful that, as challenging as it was at times, it didn't come to the worst. We must also recognize that for many people, the worst is exactly what it came to. Dr. Palangi's story, Fred Sasakamoose's story – these are two among tens of thousands. Many won't be told, and thousands across Canada can no longer be told in the first person. These are our stories, and they need to be shared and understood. It can be tempting to try to just move on, to retreat into the relative comfort of numbers without names, of statistical trends and percentages. The truth of COVID-19 is much messier and much more serious. Real people's lives were ended or disrupted, their health and livelihood damaged.

The second wave in Saskatchewan took our province from a success story to a cautionary tale. Our family watched the case counts soar as we tried our best to celebrate the holidays, taking a little extra quiet time together to reflect on the Christmas messages of sacrifice that are usually obscured among the twinkling lights.

Back to School

"Thank you @PremierScottMoe for not thinking we're essential workers, as I sit in the @PAHealthDept Vic hospital recovering from Covid-19. Get my fellow teachers vaccinated, before this happens to anyone else."[1] This was the message Vic Thunderchild posted on Twitter on April 5, 2021. Sadly, it was Vic's last public message. He passed away from COVID less than two weeks later.

Vic Thunderchild was a respected educator, guidance counsellor, and community leader in Prince Albert. A descendant of Chief Thunderchild, one of the signatories of Treaty 6, he was committed to preserving and promoting First Nations culture and language. He had helped to develop Cree language programs and was a well-known powwow dancer.

Well over six feet tall, Vic was described as a gentle giant. He spoke with humility but wasn't afraid to make his views known when they needed to be. His message came at a time when certain groups were being prioritized for access to vaccines in Saskatchewan. Despite being exposed to classrooms packed with kids where any possibility of social distancing was impossible, despite the avowed priority of keeping schools open and safe, the prioritized groups didn't include teachers.[2] The government had resisted this despite calls from the Saskatchewan Teachers' Federation and many individual educators like Vic. A week after his death, Vic's fellow teachers learned they would be given priority for protection after all. It was too late for Vic, but his advocacy may have kept other teachers safe at a time when protections were so scarce.

Perhaps nothing has been more politicized during the pandemic than the health and well-being of children. Children's lives should not be a political football, and for that reason I approach the subject with caution. At the same time, when kids have been caught in a world where their lives are disrupted and endangered by the actions of adults, the impact of that demands examination. Perhaps, when the argument comes up of "won't someone think of the children," the best test of who is acting in good faith is to see who was thinking of the children all along.

Closing the Doors

In March 2020, the consensus was clear. Schools had to close. With what was happening in Italy, Iran, and Wuhan, the risk of allowing the virus to run wild was too great. Every day kids leave their families, spend the day in a small space with dozens of kids who also have families, and then return home. It's hard to imagine a more uncontrolled site of social mixing. When Richard Halkett and Carter Mecher were developing the US pandemic response plan in the early 2000s, they brought a number of scenarios to modelling experts and asked which interventions would have the biggest impact on the spread of a respiratory virus. "When you fed into those models the question 'What happens if you do nothing but close schools and reduce the social interaction of minors by 60 percent?' They responded, slowly, but as one: that works."[3]

Closing schools works to control the virus. It doesn't work for kids. Whether it was falling behind at school, suffering from mental illness, or being put in real physical danger, the spring of 2020 made a lot of children's lives harder. It started, as it did for everyone, with fear and anxiety. Kids depend on the adults in their lives to have things under control and are incredibly sensitive to the stresses and anxieties of their grown-ups. Seeing the entire world shut down, their parents and care-givers worried and afraid, and not understanding what was happening was incredibly stressful. That's why we hosted our kids' town halls and parents' town halls, to try to share enough knowledge about COVID with local children and their parents to give them some understanding and agency in that chaotic time.

As time wore on, the initial fear turned to boredom, and for many kids to other feelings that were hard to control. They weren't playing with their friends from school or the neighbourhood or seeing the teachers, coaches, and other positive adults outside their homes. Parks and playgrounds were closed long after it was clear that was overkill. Screen time and social media use went way up, physical activity and social connection way down. Studies showed that the number of kids suffering from depression and anxiety had doubled in the first year of the pandemic.[4] For many kids, the change in routines and loss of social contacts impacted body image and relationships with food as well. The number of kids being admitted to Saskatoon's children's hospital with eating disorders tripled.[5]

Along with hurting kids' mental health, school disruptions also delayed their learning. The switch from full-time in-class instruction to a very brief online class left many children falling behind. Some couldn't attend at all because their family didn't have the tablet or computer needed to connect, or because they didn't have Wi-Fi at home or lived in rural areas without consistent internet access. That digital divide, combined with the loss of direct support from teachers and educational assistants, meant that many of the kids who needed help the most were getting next to no learning at all. Students with good home supports and an aptitude for learning may not have lost much, but those who were struggling before fell further behind, increasing the gaps within grades.

We also have to remember that not every home is a safe home at the best of times. The lack of child care options meant that many children were left alone or with a sibling, or that a parent was off work and money was tighter than ever. In Saskatchewan, where one in four children lives in poverty, many kids depend on schools for their one healthy meal of the day. Others need school to get away from home, though this question is more complicated. Being stressed out and cooped up together can increase the risk of abuse, and there were valid concerns expressed about the interference of school closures with "the detection, reporting and prevention of child abuse" as the usual early warning network of teachers and other adults outside the home was disrupted.[6] The data seem to suggest, however, that child abuse did not increase during the pandemic.[7] This may be because, along with the added stressors, there was also some relief of stress. Financial assistance and more time at home with children may have been protective factors. Many people reported "heartwarming stories about bonding with their own children,"[8] something to which Mahli and I could certainly relate. My days in the office with Abe or our outdoor adventures in the spring of 2020 are precious memories, as was the first COVID Christmas where, despite missing seeing the rest of the family, we had extra time to make things special for our boys.

As well as being tough on kids, school and child care closures are no picnic for parents. People have jobs to go to and having to figure out how to care for kids seven days a week isn't easy. We were able to make things work with our boys, but the negotiations and juggling were constant. Single parents, shift workers, and most working people were in a bind that wasn't functional. The degree to which our economy relies on kids' having somewhere to go outside the home was made more apparent than ever.

And of course, the harm done by moving to online school or closing child care spaces must be examined against the harm done if we had failed to do so. In the first twenty months of the pandemic, an estimated 5.2 million children worldwide were left orphaned due to COVID-19.[9] In the United States, 170,000 children lost a parent or caregiver to COVID in the same period.[10] During Saskatchewan's third wave, chief medical officer and ICU physician Dr. Susan Shaw told the *Saskatoon StarPhoenix* that "we're having to support young children who need to come into the intensive care unit to say goodbye to their parents. We're seeing parents that have to come into the ICU to say goodbye to their children."[11] If losing a few weeks of school is bad for a child, how much worse is having a parent coming home weak from the ICU or never coming home at all? And how incredibly tragic for parents to witness their sons and daughters dying, whether as children or adults.

We must also remember that, while the risk of serious illness for children is much lower than for adults, it is not zero, and neither is the risk of life-threatening conditions like multisystem inflammatory syndrome or potentially lifelong post-COVID symptoms. Simply put, if viral spread in schools increases community transmission, which then further increases transmission in schools, the risk to kids and adults goes up as well. There is no easy answer, no response that will do no harm at all; the policy goal must be one of balance.

If closing schools in the spring of 2020 was a reasonable choice, so was the push to see them open again in the fall. Schools are crucial for the well-being of children and for the ability of people – especially women – to get to work. The brief shutdown was justifiable at the time, but with everything we've learned since then, closing schools should clearly be a last resort. Dr. Ruth Grimes, president of the Canadian Pediatric Society, wrote to Premier Moe and Dr. Shahab at the peak of the fourth wave, urging greater action to protect children and pointing out that "children and youth suffered immeasurably from school closures and social isolation in 2020/21. We must do everything possible to ensure they can benefit from in-person learning, peer connections and social and extracurricular activities this year."[12] In a similar vein, Saskatchewan education minister Dustin Duncan said, in January 2022, that "schools should be the first to open and the last to close."[13] That is the right idea, but it further underlines the importance of doing the work to make sure those schools are safe.

What was less reasonable was the consistent messaging that this was a low-risk activity. There seemed to be a concerted effort to convince people not only that kids were at low risk from the virus but also that schools wouldn't be sites of transmission. How could we go from school closure being a very effective means of decreasing transmission to business-as-usual posing no increased risk? It's understandable given how central schools have become to the proper functioning of our society, but we needed sensible planning, not wishful thinking. This presumption of safety led to reluctance to find the right balance and to back-to-school plans that failed the grade.

Classrooms in Crisis

The problems for kids in Saskatchewan were already well known before the pandemic. More than a quarter of the children in the province live in poverty (26.1 percent), nearly ten points higher than the national average (17.7 percent).[14] The entire province could be described as a child care desert, with the lowest access to quality child care in Canada.[15] Chronic underfunding, combined with the added pressure of more students overall, more students with special needs, more students for whom English or French is a new language, more children struggling with mental health or just coming to school hungry because they're living in poverty, has led to complex, crowded classrooms. Per-student funding has been falling steadily, dropping, for example, by $344 per student in Saskatoon from 2017 to 2021.[16] In March 2020, teachers announced they would be stopping extracurricular activities as the first step to a strike. Their main demand was for a mechanism to maintain manageable classroom size and composition.[17] With the arrival of COVID that same month, there was no appetite for job action and the contract was settled without addressing class sizes. The fight was over, but the problem wasn't solved.

With a new school year on the horizon and many unanswered questions, a group of teachers and parents formed Safe Schools Saskatchewan, which emerged out of a Facebook group set up to get teachers involved in advocacy a couple of years earlier. In an interview, Saskatoon elementary school teacher Jennifer Gallays, one of the lead organizers, told me of the need for a robust plan for a safe return to school. "This COVID thing isn't going away in a few weeks. We needed a plan for what school is going to look like and it just seemed like we weren't getting anything from the government." They started by reading about places like Israel to try to learn from the experiences of countries that had already started back to school. What they'd learned had her worried:

> We can't just go back with no masks and crowded classrooms. It appears to be airborne, through smaller, finer respiratory droplets. Schools often don't have good ventilation; some don't have opening windows and we pack a bunch of kids into there. So, these things they were telling us to do at that point, you know, the three C's of avoid crowded spaces, close contact, and closed spaces, well ... that's a school, that's a classroom!

As an opposition, we worked with teachers and public health experts to outline key elements of a safe back-to-school plan, including dedicated transition funds, smaller class sizes, increased testing and tracing capacity, clear communications on outbreaks, availability of online learning as an option or if required due to outbreaks, and clear guidance and provision of PPE.[18] Instead, while other provinces were mandating mask use in preparation for a second wave, the Saskatchewan plan focused on staggered lunch hours and promoting "air high fives" over hugging. This was the direct result of the downplaying of risks to kids and led to poor choices in the design of those eventual back-to-school plans. Masks, which are one of the least disruptive and most easily tolerated measures, were only reluctantly and belatedly introduced. When they were, they were accompanied by odd exceptions, like the advice that kids didn't need to mask if they were facing forward at their desks. Kids don't stay facing forward and viruses that are airborne (which SARS-CoV-2 was well-known to be by the time schools returned in the fall) don't raise their hands and ask permission to circulate through the room. Just like the idea of social distancing in an overcrowded Grade 3 classroom, that sort of recommendation seemed to come from someone who hadn't set foot in a school for decades.

The plan was widely panned by teachers and parents. Saskatoon high school student Kiera Krogstad wrote: "I know the teachers and staff at my school will try their best to keep us safe, but without the right support and funding, their hands are tied. The adults have control here and they are supposed to keep us safe, but it seems like they don't even care about us." Protests, organized in part by Safe Schools Saskatchewan, were held outside the office of then education minister Gord Wyant. The negative public response sent the Saskatchewan Party back to the drawing board, releasing a new plan two weeks later that added new funding and delayed the start of the school year by a week, but remained unclear on masking and offered nothing regarding improved ventilation as recommended by the federal government.[19]

Within days of schools opening, there were outbreaks at multiple high schools. Masks in schools came weeks after the province-wide indoor mask mandate was introduced. This baffled Jennifer Gallays: "It was just mind-boggling to us that society has these health mandates, but they don't apply at all to school? Have you been in a school lately? We're teaching kids that are as big as us and you're trying to tell us they're not spreading the virus? It just felt like a lot of gaslighting." By the middle of the second wave in November, over twenty schools had active outbreaks. Throughout the period, case counts were being tracked and publicly shared; the under-nineteen age group had the second highest rates of infection, and a quarter of those were understood to be transmitted within the schools.[20] Along with the spread within schools, the failure to keep community transmission low meant that the stated mission of keeping schools open also failed. Many families, ours included, dealt with the scramble of figuring out what do when an outbreak closed their child's classroom for a week or ten days. In the second, third, and fifth waves, Regina public schools were forced to close their doors outright, either because of elevated risk or because there were so many teachers off sick that they couldn't staff their classrooms.[21] It was hard to comprehend why, as the virus spread wildly, we were keeping restaurants and bars open and closing schools.

More kids became severely ill as time went on. Our high rates of illness and low rates of vaccination are what prompted Dr. Grimes's letter calling for greater action to protect children and their in-school learning.[22] As of October 2021, 124 kids had been admitted to hospital, 20 of those to the ICU.[23] In one week that month, 17 children had COVID infections serious enough to be admitted to hospital. At that time, we learned that 3 children under twelve had already died in the province, accounting for 16 percent of the child deaths in Canada, the highest per capita child death rate in the country. These are not huge numbers but, as Mahli – who had presented the updated child hospitalization and mortality data at a physicians' town hall – told the *StarPhoenix*, "kids as a population do not die in large numbers, and any pediatric death is a devastating event that needs to be considered carefully and the events and policies leading to it carefully analyzed."[24]

In fall 2022, Canada was experiencing a wave of child hospitalizations. Pediatric wards saw double or triple their usual rates of admission as they became swamped with what was referred to as a "triple-demic" of influenza, respiratory syncytial virus (RSV), and COVID.[25] The chief of staff at Ottawa's Children's Hospital called for a return to masking to help stem the tide.[26] This challenged the idea that COVID was a minor concern for kids. With under 7 percent of children under five having received their COVID vaccine at the time,[27] the hyper-politicization of children's vaccines had proven to be foolish as we leave kids unprotected from short- and long-term problems. Alongside the health problems, the *Pedianomics* report released by Children First Canada in May 2023 indicated that the triple-demic cost the Canadian economy $60 million due to parents missing work.

Catching Up

The impact on mental health and learning has left an enormous amount of work to help kids catch up to their peers. Pre-existing gaps between First Nations and Métis children, children of newcomers, and the rest of the population have worsened, as have gaps resulting from differences in socio-economic status.

Jennifer Gallays has been teaching for over twenty years. She says the gaps have widened more than she's ever seen:

> I taught online all last year. I started out with about thirty-three kids in my online class. Three had intensive needs, so they had a full-time educational assistant in the classroom but not online. I had four to eight kids, depending on what point in the year, that were English as an Additional Language, they had support in a physical classroom, they didn't have support online.

Kids in French immersion fell behind in language learning, younger kids lost ground in reading. Many children in more challenging social situations left school and didn't return.

Now that kids are back in class and having to catch up, they need more help than before. They need smaller class sizes and one-on-one attention more than ever. Jennifer describes what a difference those numbers make. "If I have a class of 21 kids, I can be the support for all those kids. In the last number of years I've had 28, 30, 32, 33, and with intense needs." At a time like this, one might expect to see a greater investment in education. Unfortunately, Saskatchewan saw the opposite, with the 2022 budget again falling short of the cost of inflation and growing student enrolment. Instead of bringing in more people to help kids catch up, divisions across the province were having to cut staff positions. The Cornerstone School Division in Southeast Saskatchewan cut twenty-one teachers and eleven support staff. Saskatoon Public Schools eliminated thirteen full-time positions in elementary schools and seven in high schools, and had to start charging families for lunchtime supervision.[28]

The only interest conservative governments seem to be taking in Canadian schools is insisting that they not take action to protect kids' health. In Alberta, Minister of Education Adriana Grange was found to have interfered with public health decision-making in February 2022 after insisting that schools in her province drop their mask mandates.[29] The same month, Dustin Duncan, Saskatchewan's education minister, would follow Alberta's lead by ordering all school divisions to drop all public health measures, including masking.[30] When the Ontario Principals' Council and the Children's Health Coalition called for continued masking in March 2022, the province refused.[31]

We hear a lot about burnout in the health professions. With health teams asked to step up and put their health on the line after years of cuts and understaffing, many people are thinking about leaving. The same elements are at play in our schools. A study in British Columbia reported that 80 percent of teachers were struggling with their mental health and two in five were more likely to leave the profession than before the pandemic.[32] In Alberta over a third of teachers surveyed by the Alberta Teachers' Association said they likely wouldn't be in the classroom in five years.[33] In Saskatchewan 40 percent of teachers surveyed in 2019 reported having considered quitting due to burnout,[34] and that was before the pandemic. We saw people retiring early rather than working as substitutes, contributing to teacher shortages in 2021. Jennifer Gallays worries about the effect on new teachers coming into the profession: "As for a mass-exodus, I worry about that happening, and it's not on the back-end where people are retiring, it's the front," as either those who might be considering teaching or those who are staring down the prospect of a long and challenging career find themselves discouraged and looking for other options.

Treating kids well is the right thing to do for them and for all of us. Our long-term health and well-being depend upon giving the young people in our world the opportunity to grow and to thrive. Education is a key social determinant at any time and is crucial to resilience in times of trouble. Those who would reduce the quality of public schools to save money or cut education taxes to stimulate the economy have an incredibly short-sighted and narrow vision of what makes an economy function. Which returns me to my initial point. In times when public debate focuses on what's good for children, it's helpful to ask whether the people having the debate have been acting in the best interests of children to begin with.

With the growing rates of respiratory illness and the unknown future impact of repeated COVID infections on children, it is not too late to act to protect kids. This includes measures such as transparent sharing of information on outbreaks, increased ventilation, including the use of HEPA filtration, and masking in periods or regions where risk is high.[35] More importantly in the long-term, the best protection for our kids is an educational system that is well resourced. Decreasing the level of stress by properly supporting teachers, making sure classes aren't overcrowded, and funding the supports kids need to catch up after a difficult time is the best way to ensure healthy children this year and for a lifetime to come. How we provide for kids today will make all the difference in whether we have a healthy future tomorrow.

Respecting Our Elders

When Corey Atkinson saw his dad's number on his phone, he felt a sinking feeling in his stomach. He'd seen the news a few days earlier that there was an outbreak at Parkside Extendicare, the long-term care (LTC) home in Regina where his mother, Myrna, was living. He knew what COVID had done in care homes in Quebec and Ontario and understood immediately that his family was in for hard times.

Canada's first wave was marked by deadly outbreaks among residents and staff in LTC homes. More than 5,000 Canadian seniors living in congregate settings lost their lives in 840 COVID-19 outbreaks in the spring of 2020. This accounted for over 80 percent of Canada's COVID deaths at the time, a rate more than twice the OECD average.[1] In that period, seventy-four times as many elderly adults died from COVID-19 in LTC than outside. In Ontario, the Canadian Armed Forces took over five homes with particularly bad outbreaks, eventually releasing a scathing report that identified numerous problems, including staff moving from room to room without changing PPE, rooming of COVID-positive patients with uninfected residents, and a consistent lack of adequate staffing.[2]

The military's revelations were shocking at the time, but the truth is short-staffing and inadequate care were the norm before and have been since in care homes across Canada. *Globe and Mail* health columnist André Picard puts it starkly: "Eldercare in this country is so disorganized and so poorly regulated, the staffing so inadequate, the accountability so non-existent and ageism so rampant, there seems to be no limit to what care homes can get away with."[3] We've become so accustomed to the systemic neglect of Canadian seniors that it appears no one thought twice about the harm headed their way. The first-wave focus was so heavily on hospitals and community transmission that an entire segment of our society – people packed into tight, shared quarters and with the least reserve to fight infection – was completely ignored. This clearly reflects the long-standing problems in long-term care and the general pandemic unpreparedness that left the country scrambling so badly that we missed such a key and pressing risk.

It also brings to light the ageism that informed people's attitudes and comments about who was at risk and who was an "acceptable loss."[4] For example, then Alberta premier Jason Kenney said in the Alberta legislature in June 2020 that "the average age of death from COVID in Alberta is eighty-three and I remind the house that the average life expectancy in the province is age eighty-two," and referred to the pandemic as an "influenza that does not generally threaten life apart from the most elderly."[5] Along with being an ugly dismissal of the value of elderly lives, this would prove to be a premature assessment of the age risk. At 47 percent, Kenney's Alberta would wind up not far behind Saskatchewan's nation-leading 55 percent of COVID deaths occurring in those under age eighty.[6]

Worse than the inaccuracy is the disturbing level of comfort with the premature demise of older people displayed in this characterization of the pandemic. It was a shockingly common notion throughout the pandemic, and one that brought to mind Paul Farmer's famous phrase, "the idea that some lives matter less is the root of all that is wrong with the world."[7] Dr. Theresa Tam, Canada's chief public health officer said, "We failed the most vulnerable people in our society."[8] Interviewed by CTV, Tam reflected: "I think the tragedy and the massive lesson learned for everyone in Canada is that we were at every level, not able to protect our seniors, particularly those in LTC homes." She went on to remark that "even worse is that in that second wave, as we warned of the resurgence, there was a repeat of the huge impact on that population."[9]

Long-Term Problem

In the fall of 2020, Scott Moe said what a good thing it was that, unlike other provinces, Saskatchewan had been spared major problems in LTC. And he was right, that good fortune was something to be proud of. Having seen what had happened elsewhere, our provincial government could have made the changes and investment needed to keep it that way. We had the heads-up that everyone else had missed, the chance to learn from the mistakes of others instead of insisting on making our own. Most of the deaths in LTC elsewhere in the country had occurred in the first month of the pandemic, while our understanding of testing and transmission was much more limited. In the meantime, we'd seen models of how to do better. For example, British Columbia took what Health Minister Adrian Dix called a "whole of sector approach," turning their experience from earlier outbreaks into an approach where they quickly introduced cohorting so that workers weren't moving between homes, increased infection control standards, brought in extra payment to support lost hours and financial help when people needed to be off work, and introduced aggressive contact tracing and testing in response to suspected outbreaks.[10]

In Saskatchewan, we had the time and resources to staff up in LTC, to increase our testing and tracing capacity, to learn from the best. Instead, the Saskatchewan Party chose magical thinking. The results were disastrous.

My mother, Lea Meili, trained and then practised as a registered nurse at Providence Hospital in Moose Jaw. She took a few years off work to stay on the farm and raise my brothers and me to school age. She then returned to practice at Extendicare in Moose Jaw, working on the floor for seven years, for ten as an RN and assistant director of care, and then going on to be administrator for the final eight years of her career. As a kid, I would go and chat with residents in the activity room while waiting for her to get off work, and later would visit frequently when two of my grandparents spent their final days in that same home. I witnessed the care my mother carried for the residents, their families, and the staff, and the way those staff went to extremes to make sure residents were given not just a place to stay but a safe and loving home.

This is the work ethic and philosophy of those who serve in LTC. The staff adopts the residents as extended family. But they can't work miracles, they can't create something out of nothing. When they are overworked and underpaid, mistakes get made. When the regulations and resources that should be in place to support them in their work are missing, people get hurt. Tragically, those frontline care workers are constantly put in situations where all the goodwill in the world can't overcome the lack of resources. The mistreatment of seniors is systemic neglect and an example of what Paul Farmer called structural violence.

Dr. Thomas Hadjistavropoulos, director of the Centre on Aging and Health at the University of Regina, told the *Leader-Post:* "COVID has not caused the problems that we're facing, COVID has exposed the problems that have already been there."[11] He's right, though perhaps "re-exposed" would have been the better phrase. In 2014, then leader of the Opposition Cam Broten raised the story of Margaret Warholm, a seventy-four-year-old resident of a Regina care home who had died after suffering from malnutrition and a bedsore that covered her entire back.[12] On dozens of occasions, Broten highlighted stories like Margaret's to expose the dangerous conditions in LTC and call on the government to take action.

Report after report from the provincial ombudsman and other reviewers supported Broten's conclusions, revealing overcrowding, poor ventilation, and insufficient staffing in seniors' homes in Saskatchewan. There are no minimum standards for baths, staffing levels, or minimum hours of care per resident. Prior to 2011, homes were required to have sufficient staff to provide two hours of care per day to each resident, but that requirement was eliminated by the Sask Party government in 2011. In my conversations with LTC workers, they describe often having less than fifteen minutes a day to help residents with washing, dressing, and mealtimes, much less than the over three hours per resident legislated in other provinces. These problems have been raised repeatedly in our legislature and in the media, but the province chose not to make the changes necessary to provide dignified care and keep people safe. Hundreds of families are now grieving the entirely preventable loss of a loved one as a result. Many more are worried today about the ongoing troubles for current residents, or desperately trying to avoid placing an aging family member in LTC but are unable to find adequate home care supports to make that possible. Years of intentional underinvestment, of corporate ownership and government oversight ignoring call bell after call bell, set the stage for Saskatchewan's biggest COVID-19 tragedy: the Parkside Extendicare outbreak.

Danger in Care

Myrna Atkinson was born in Balcarres in 1954 and grew up on a farm near Broadview, not far from her mother's home reserve of Cowessess First Nation. When she graduated from high school, she joined the military and met her husband, Steve, in basic training in Ontario. After a few postings, including several years in Moose Jaw, they settled in Regina. Steve continued in the military, but Myrna retired when their son Corey was born, working at Canadian Tire, Sears, and later with the provincial Information Services Corporation.

Her health began to deteriorate early on. She suffered from chronic renal failure and eventually needed a kidney transplant. She had severe back troubles, which limited her mobility to the point that there were several episodes where she couldn't walk at all. After back surgery in 2014, she wasn't recovering as well as expected and it was discovered she had chronic leukemia. After two or three years of exhausting struggle at home, where she needed daily therapy just to be able to walk, she ended up spending several weeks in the Regina Pasqua hospital. Myrna was stuck in the all-too-common limbo of being too unwell to go home, not sick enough to be admitted, but having nowhere else to go.

This is a chronic problem in our hospitals, where the lack of home care and LTC capacity leaves entire wards of patients "waiting for placement" for months on end. It costs $100 a day to support a long-term care eligible senior in their own home, $200 a day in a long-term care facility. In hospital, that cost rises to $750 a day.[13] It's an enormous added cost for an inferior experience, as even the most limited of care homes offers a more peaceful environment and more opportunities to socialize than a hospital room.

This warehousing of seniors in hospital wards also creates a chain reaction in the health care system. The "bed block" of occupied rooms leaves newly admitted patients in emergency rooms and hallways, making it impossible to receive all the patients who need care, leaving ambulances lined up in the parking lot and people at home unable to get emergency care. It becomes clear why patients, families, and staff are keen to find somewhere, anywhere else to go, often accepting something less than ideal just to get away from the hospital.

That's how Myrna came to live at Parkside in late 2019, much to the disappointment of her family. When asked about this move, Corey said, "We weren't crazy about it, to be honest." They had hoped she could be in a place with her own room, but instead she was one of four residents to a room. "They were packed in like sardines," he said. "It wasn't safe." These four-bed rooms had been flagged as out of step with current standards of care, including by then minister of health Dustin Duncan as far back as 2013.[14]

Despite all of these health problems, Myrna made the best of her new home. At sixty-six, despite her serious health problems, she had energy for life. She looked forward to visits from her husband, son, and grandchildren, even when COVID came and those visits had to be done through a fence in the yard. The loss of in-person visits was not only a source of isolation for residents, though that was of course a serious hardship. One of the ways of keeping staffing levels of LTC homes so low is by depending on family members to assist with the daily care of residents, helping with dressing, brushing teeth, and other time-consuming tasks. The loss of those extra hands highlighted the short-staffing and contributed to the oversights that would occur in the months ahead.

Corey, a broadcast journalist in Regina, was worried about his mother that fall. She told him she'd be wheeled out into the yard long before they arrived for their scheduled visits, and left waiting long after they'd gone. She'd been weaker and more tired since she'd caught a skin infection called scabies during an outbreak that fall. Parkside Extendicare was well known for its problems with infectious disease management. For example, from January to July 2020 the facility saw thirteen infectious outbreaks, including a gastrointestinal virus, scabies, and eleven respiratory viruses.[15] When Corey heard of the COVID outbreak, he knew Myrna was in real danger. He thought of how fast the virus spread, of how she was immunocompromised from her leukemia treatment, and of that packed four-bed room.

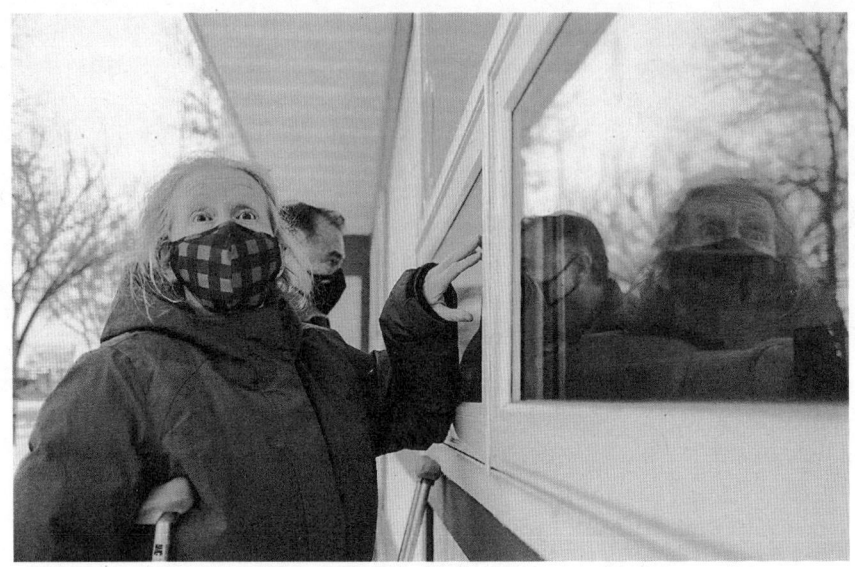

Window visit. Pam Moore speaks about her mother,
Joan Moore, who had recently tested positive for COVID-19,
while husband Rob Coleman looks on at the Extendicare Parkside
care home. December 2020 | *Michael Bell, Regina Leader-Post*

The danger came. Corey got a call from his dad on November 21 – his parents' forty-fifth wedding anniversary – that his mom had contracted COVID and was going to the hospital. A few days later she was in the ICU. Corey knew how serious the disease was and that in Myrna's condition she couldn't handle a long ICU stay. He started to prepare himself for the fact that this could be the end. He remembers waiting for his dad in the hospital parking lot, agonizingly close to where his mother lay dying but unable to go see her. He felt helpless, knowing that someone he loved and cared about was in such a desperate situation and that he couldn't be there for her to see him, to know that he was there for her.

Myrna died on December 4 without Corey having a chance to even hold her hand and say goodbye. This left him feeling angry, feeling like something had been taken from him. He was angry that the government saw what had happened in Ontario and Quebec and hadn't learned anything. That they'd seen so many infectious disease outbreaks in Parkside and hadn't changed a thing to keep people safe. Angry that his mom was gone, her life cut short earlier than it needed to be, and that because of the pandemic the family could only hold a Zoom conference instead of a funeral.

The Extendicare Parkside Outbreak

Myrna was the second resident to lose her life to COVID-19 at Parkside in what would turn out to be a tragic winter. It started on November 11, 2020, when a care worker at the facility developed a cough and headache and felt dizzy. The next day they lost their sense of smell. They had followed the rules, wearing masks in public places and when working with residents. Staff were not required to mask during breaks, and residents did not wear masks inside or outside their rooms. Staff also frequently carpooled to work and did not mask in shared vehicles. Between November 9, when they would have been positive but asymptomatic, and getting a positive COVID-19 test on November 20, this staff member worked eleven shifts in the home. Two more staff members developed symptoms the following week.

On the morning of November 17, a resident was found slumped and unconscious in their wheelchair and was helped into bed. At the time their oxygen saturation (sats) was 94 percent. By evening, their breath had become "gurgly" and their sats were in the sixties. The resident was taken to hospital by ambulance, and, by two the next morning, had died from complications of COVID-19, the first Parkside resident to test positive and die from COVID.

The number of positive cases would rise to seventeen residents and seven staff a week later, and the facility started to isolate residents into positive and non-positive cohorts. The sheer number of cases and the lack of space made this a chaotic process, with staff and residents moving between positive and non-positive areas, likely contributing to the spread of the virus. By December 6, there were ninety positive residents and forty-five positive staff, the Regina Fire Department had to be called in to provide staffing support, and twenty-five COVID-negative residents were moved to another care home in the city. Most of these residents would go on to test positive despite that move, though the outbreak did not spread into the Pioneer Village home that hosted them.[16]

The Saskatchewan Health Authority then realized the situation was too severe for Extendicare to continue to handle it. They declared the outbreak an emergency, took over management, and put out a call to mobilize staff from across the health system. One staff member spoke anonymously to the CBC, saying that "it was a war zone." "We were losing people every day," he said. "It was unimaginable, the conditions inside. They were so short-staffed."[17] The death count continued to climb, with one or more deaths recorded nearly every day from the beginning of December into the New Year.

By the time the outbreak was declared over on January 21, 2021, 136 staff members and all but 4 of 198 residents had tested positive for the virus. Forty-two of those positive residents died, 39 from COVID-19 and another 3 reportedly from other causes, making it by far the deadliest outbreak in the province.

Toward the end of the outbreak, the NDP opposition introduced a motion calling for an independent inquiry into the Parkside outbreak.[18] The government chose to defeat that motion in the house, although two weeks later seniors minister Everett Hindley called on Mary McFadyen, then provincial ombudsman, to investigate the actions of Extendicare during the outbreak.[19] She agreed, but rejected the minister's limitation of her investigation to the actions of Extendicare, insisting on examining the role of the Saskatchewan Health Authority and the Ministry of Health as well.[20]

Parkside Extendicare was a pile of dried kindling, ready to go up in flames. Choices made by corporate and government leadership served as lighter fluid. The virus was only the spark. The conditions and choices that created that level of danger, as informed by the ombudsman's investigation, media coverage, and staff statements, can be broken down into three major categories: structure and planning, staff support, and accountability. Looking back now, it's clear there were many alarm bells that should have been rung, others that rang loudly only to be ignored. Hopefully, by examining how this tragedy occurred in one of so many homes across Canada that were ravaged by outbreaks, we can learn something about how to better protect the most vulnerable and support the frontline staff charged with their care.

Profit before People

At a time when so much emphasis was being placed on social distancing, here was a facility where four seniors, people who, through either underlying illness or just the reality of waning immunity with age, were high-risk by definition, shared a small and crowded room. At the time of the outbreak, Parkside Extendicare had twelve single rooms, forty two-bed rooms, and thirty-four four-bed rooms. That's 136 residents in four-bed rooms, breathing the same air, using the same washroom, and being cared for by staff moving from room to room. And everyone in a position to do something about it was fully aware of the problem.

The class action lawsuit filed against Extendicare by the families of the victims of the outbreak pointed out that building standards for new nursing homes have not allowed four-person rooms since 1999.[21] Parkside, which had been built in the 1960s, was well known to be out of date. A report in 2011 highlighted, among other shortcomings, the infection control issues associated with having four residents to a room.[22] The Sask Party approved a replacement for the home in 2012 at Extendicare's request, but a decade of promises later, nothing had been done.

Families of residents shared their distress at leaving loved ones in a rundown building with cluttered hallways, peeling paint on the walls, and a strong smell throughout.[23] A 2019 health authority report described Parkside's status as we headed into the pandemic: "The facility is old and in need of replacement due to pending infrastructure and large system (HVAC) failures. The current design with a large number of 4-bed rooms does not meet current standards of care or resident and family expectations for a home environment."[24] As the ombudsman pointed out in her 2021 report *Caring in Crisis,* it is crystal-clear that both Extendicare and the health authority were fully aware of the problems at Parkside prior to the pandemic. McFadyen also found that Extendicare could and should have done away with four-bed rooms, as demonstrated by their choice to eliminate four-bed rooms after the outbreak. But they didn't. Once the pandemic arrived, there were emails and meetings about the problem. There was not, however, any action.

Why? Because they were arguing about money. Extendicare wouldn't make any changes without assurances that they would not lose out financially. An email from the company's regional director to the health authority in August 2020 said that "any bed reduction strategy would need to be supported with funding to ensure as an organization, we don't experience any financial risk and are 'kept whole'" and emphasized the long-term replacement of the home over the immediate danger to residents. Extendicare wasn't wrong that this would be costly for them, and the health authority likely had legitimate constraints in addressing those costs, but these are people's lives we're talking about here. It is reminiscent of the Jordan's Principle concept from the world of First Nations children's welfare, and the idea is the same: when the well-being of vulnerable people is at risk, get them safe first, then figure out who pays for it. Instead, Extendicare and the SHA argued, first for a decade while the discomfort of residents was real but the risks more abstract, and then for months when danger was right outside the door. They argued over money and people died as a result.

The ability to cohort staff to Extendicare was impacted by their being separate from the larger pool of employees in public facilities. This resulted in Parkside being even more understaffed than usual, a chronic problem at a facility that had a hard time attracting staff. When the outbreak hit, this meant that staff were moving between the rooms of those who were COVID-positive or working in positive and negative wings of the care home in the same shift. This also meant that staff was unable to properly supervise residents, meaning infected patients with dementia could wander into other rooms.

Attempts to move residents were described by workers as "a whole lot of chaos," as "negative residents were sitting in the hallways while we're trying to get rooms cleaned."[25] There were also too few cleaning staff available to thoroughly clean the rooms that had housed positive residents. Add to this the failure to social-distance residents at mealtimes and staff at breaks, and you have a situation where a failure to plan effectively led to increased transmission of the virus.

On top of the shortage of in-house care staff, a government decision reduced the amount of medical support to the facility. In April 2020, in a move that is very hard to reconcile with what was happening at the time, compensation rules were changed so that physicians could bill for visits to LTC homes only every fourteen days rather than once a week as previously. This meant a cut of 50 percent to doctors' fees for visits and a financial decision by the government to decrease the amount of medical service provided for seniors in care, a very strange choice in general but especially just as the pandemic was starting.[26] Two doctors did visit Parkside on December 2, nearly two weeks after the outbreak was declared. They raised the alarm, with one writing to the health authority: "Why can't we stop the spread? 80 patients is a disaster! Is it PPE, is it staff fatigue, we need people on the ground to figure it out. The staff is just tired and surviving. Patients are dying and more without a doubt will die."[27] The next day more supports were brought in. Would it have taken as long if doctors were on-site more often?

Like many workplaces, Parkside put in place reasonable questionnaires and temperature checks, but these were haphazardly enforced.[28] To Extendicare national's credit, however, they did try to learn from the experience in Ontario and requested routine testing of their LTC staff. Extendicare felt this would have prevented the spread from the first staff member, who wasn't tested for over a week after presenting with symptoms,[29] along with other cases. The Ministry of Health rejected this idea and refused to perform weekly testing on staff.[30]

A stranger approach from Extendicare was their reluctance to provide proper PPE for staff. Staff were given a single mask per day and a paper bag to store it in when not in use, and were discouraged from requesting more. This was contrary to the provincial guidelines that masks should be discarded at breaks and at the end of the shift, a minimum of four masks per day. The regional management felt it didn't have to follow the provincial rules. Further to this, Extendicare management also refused to enforce the provincial public health rules requiring that residents be masked when outside their rooms, despite this being a requirement for over a month. The regional director even sent an email complaining about this requirement on December 23, after nearly every resident of the facility had been infected and over thirty had already lost their lives.

Parkside thought it could do its own thing. As of April 29, 2020, it was the only facility in the province that didn't complete the COVID-19 readiness checklist from the provincial pandemic plan, and it still hadn't by October 26, days before the outbreak began. Extendicare was viewed – both by provincial bodies and by the company itself – as a private entity that wasn't required to follow provincial directions or standards. Per the ombudsman's report, "because Extendicare is an independent company, they [the SHA] did not have the authority to require it to comply with the Authority's continuous masking protocols and guidelines – even though they knew it was not complying with them. Instead, they believed they could only 'encourage' it to comply."[31] Given that Extendicare chose to do less to protect residents because of this belief, it amounts to a lower class of seniors' home where residents and their families are expected to accept subpar care because of private ownership. This is unfair to residents and to the staff that care for them, and in the case of the fall 2020 outbreak, that inferior quality of service was a deadly disparity.

A Broken System

This may all seem very specific to one facility or to one province, but the truth is that private, for-profit care homes have been known to provide lower quality care for years, in Canada and around the world. A 2009 study of the quality of care in for-profit versus not-for-profit care homes showed lower staffing levels, more pressure ulcers, and more frequent use of physical restraints at for-profit homes.[32] This was a follow-up to an earlier study that demonstrated that private for-profit hospitals were associated with a statistically significant increase in the risk of death.[33]

The reason for this disparity is simple, as York University professor and LTC researcher Pat Armstrong told the *Toronto Star:* "Some of the money is going to go for profits. And in order to get the profits, they have to cut back in some areas."[34] COVID-19 made the damage from those shortcuts so much clearer. A report from the Ontario Science Table showed that the two biggest risk factors for a large LTC COVID outbreak were for-profit status and crowding.[35] For-profit care homes had 78 percent more deaths than public or not-for-profit.[36] These homes had chain ownership and tended to be, like Parkside, older buildings that fall short of current standards.

In Saskatchewan, the majority of deaths were in private care as well. As of October 2021, 154 people had died in LTC. Sixty-two of those deaths were in private, not-for-profit homes (often run by faith-based organizations or municipalities). Forty-five were in private, for-profit homes. That latter number is particularly high, given that the only for-profit homes in Saskatchewan are the five run by Extendicare. That means nearly a third of deaths happened in facilities that make up just over 5 percent of the total beds.

Prior to the release of the ombudsman's report that further strengthened the rationale for change, I called for the removal of Extendicare as an operator of care homes in the province. Extendicare owns and operates five homes, three in Regina, one in Moose Jaw, and one in Saskatoon, all of which saw outbreaks of various levels of severity. We did receive pushback from some Extendicare employees for making that call. That's understandable; it can be very hard to separate criticism of the company from their role as care workers in the Extendicare homes. It's important to again emphasize that the company, and the government that should be regulating its actions, let everyone down, including the dedicated staff who wanted to do better. I know how hard the staff and leadership within those facilities work to provide care for the residents. They give it their all and have, especially at Parkside, been through a terrible experience, putting themselves in danger as they've dealt with the tragedy of losing so many of their residents. For their sake and the sake of the residents they serve, we need to have the best model of care, and it's clear that's not for-profit care.

After continued pressure, the province finally capitulated and announced, in October 2021, that the Saskatchewan Health Authority would take over the five Extendicare homes, hopefully ending for-profit seniors' care in Saskatchewan for good. The issue has not been entirely resolved yet, as Extendicare still operates these homes and, in September 2022, fourteen staff and every single resident of the forty-six-bed Elmview Extendicare in Regina contracted COVID. Three residents died during the outbreak.[37]

Eliminating for-profit care is a good start, but it's not the whole story by any means. It's also much easier to do in Saskatchewan, where the private, for-profit sector plays a much smaller role. The truth is, while the public sector does better, it doesn't necessarily do well. Issues of understaffing and poor-quality care are sector-wide, in small homes and large. The National Institute on Ageing and the Canadian Medical Association partnered on a report called *Pandemic Perspectives on Long-Term Care*. They described how "the pandemic has exposed the persistent gaps in funding, capacity and expertise across Canada's LTC systems and their inability to protect residents."[38] No wonder, then, as the surveys done for that report showed, that 86 percent of respondents over age sixty-five believed care home staff were underpaid, 91 percent believed homes were understaffed, and a full 96 percent of those seniors would do anything to avoid moving into LTC.

As an internal report on seniors' homes from Revera Inc., which is at least partially owned by Extendicare, succinctly described, "COVID-19 not only exposed cracks within the sector, but also the broken links between it and the system as a whole."[39] With even the companies behind some of the worst outbreaks acknowledging there are major problems in the sector, the question now is, if COVID revealed the problems, how can our experience of the last two years also shine a light on solutions?

"As we rebuild society and the economy, we have an opportunity to do things differently, to do them better. Elders have borne the brunt of the COVID-19 pandemic, and they should be the greatest beneficiaries as we come out the other side ... It's long past time for the neglect to end."[40] This is the conclusion reached by André Picard in his mid-pandemic book *Neglected No More: The Urgent Need to Improve the Lives of Canada's Elders in the Wake of a Pandemic.*[41] This concise, accessible work is required reading for anyone trying to imagine a better approach to the mess that is seniors' care in Canada, or for those considering the aging options for themselves and their families.

The first thing to note is that our task is not to fix LTC, or at least not to fix LTC alone. The temptation will be to try to improve the institutional model we have, perhaps even build more of the same. That would be a tremendous failure. Yes, we need to improve the quality of institutional care. We also have to take more of the needed care out of institutions.

For the care homes themselves, the first step is to end the role of for-profit LTC providers. As Tamara Daly, political economist and health services researcher at York University in Toronto, told Picard, "the research is clear on this: there is no doubt that reducing profit-taking would improve care, and we really need to improve care."[42] These facilities must integrate with the public health care system, allowing greater communication and coordination between care at home, in acute settings, and in LTC. We also need to ensure that existing buildings are safe, addressing the ventilation and crowding issues that contributed to deadly COVID outbreaks. When discussing new or replacement facilities, "we need to stop with the elder apartheid and integrate care homes into the community. Facilities should be shared with daycares and schools."[43] Community integration can help end the stigma associated with aging and help reduce the isolation that accelerates decline.

Whether in private, not-for-profit, or public facilities, we then need to fix the chronic understaffing. Minimum standards of care and resident-to-staff ratios are a must. Training a new generation of care workers will bring needed new jobs and help support the exhausted existing workforce. The federal government has said it will make a major investment in improving LTC but may tie those funds to national standards.[44] As someone who was a provincial politician, it is supposed to be my reflex response to resist any such imposition and demand full control of the funds. Unfortunately, I've witnessed what happens. Provinces do take the money and run, and we have, in health accord after health accord, little to show for billions used to backfill other parts of provincial budgets instead of buying real reform. I also recognize it will be challenging to reach a national agreement because of that reflex resistance, and that any real action on this file will demand initiative on the part of provincial leaders. Across the country, they have failed us on this file for decades. We can only hope that the pandemic will be impetus enough to end the neglect.

Most importantly, we need to reimagine aging in place. "Building institutional beds is extremely costly. Affordable housing combined with home care services is far more cost-effective and more humane."[45] Somewhere between 20 and 50 percent of current LTC residents could be cared for at home, representing enormous savings and a greatly preferred experience.[46] As a nation, we spend six dollars in LTC for every dollar spent on home care.[47] Correcting that imbalance will require some new thinking. It demands staffing up and expanding the services available through home care, but that's not all. "The main reason elders are driven out of their homes is not illness but everyday barriers to getting around in the community."[48] Programs to help seniors "age-proof" their home, improved public transit, and accessible public spaces can make living in community safer. Lastly, we need to support the informal caregivers. There are some existing tax credit programs to offset lost income for those who choose to provide care to a loved one at home. These need to be enhanced but also expanded to provide support to low-income caregivers. Only in Nova Scotia are these families eligible for a monthly benefit.[49] "This lack of financial support means that people end up in LTC earlier, even if they have family members who are willing to provide care at home."[50]

These are some of the key principles to bring to a consideration of the future of care of the elderly in Canada. We can't bring back Myrna Atkinson or any of the other thousands of seniors lost across the country during COVID-19. We can honour their memory by allowing this tragedy to open our eyes to the depths of the problem. We can commit to ensuring that our parents and grandparents are able to age with the safety and dignity that we would want for ourselves.

Third Wave

At this point, it doesn't matter whether
you call it the plague or growing pains. All that
matters is that you stop it killing half the town.

– Albert Camus, *The Plague*

Total cases in Canada	509,978
Total cases in Saskatchewan	24,624
Deaths from COVID in Canada	2,927
Deaths from COVID in Saskatchewan	233

Provincial Public Health Measures

February 9, 2021	Vaccine rollout plan announced
March 9, 2021	Household bubbles can be extended to ten people and three households, places of worship can operate at 30 percent capacity
March 18, 2021	Three-hour vaccination leave announced
March 23, 2021	All private indoor gatherings in Regina are prohibited; travel not recommended to and from Regina

Miracles and Mudholes

In the summer between my second and third years of medical school, I travelled to Mozambique with my friend Paul Olszynski, who now practises as an emergency room physician in Saskatoon. We spent two months studying and working in a rural hospital in Massinga, a small town in Inhambane Province, as part of the University of Saskatchewan's Training for Health Renewal Program led by Drs. Gerri and Murray Dickson. This program trained Mozambican health workers to become trainers of the next generation, as well as offering introductory programs for various levels of health workers. Paul and I spent our days at the hospital across the road, rounding in the in-patient wards and assisting in the *banco de socorro* (Portuguese for "emergency room"), and our nights helping out with car accidents and emergency deliveries.

Once or twice a week, we'd pile into the back of a pickup with students and local public health staff and drive anywhere from twenty to a hundred kilometres into the countryside for *brigadas movéis* (mobile brigades). There were some small villages, but for the most part the communities consisted of a series of small family compounds by mango and tangerine trees and fields of manioc or maize. The occasional wealthier family had a house made from cement or zinc sheets, but most had walls and roofs of woven palm fronds. We would pull up into a clearing and hang two portable scales from tree branches. The scales had hooks on the bottom where we would attach a sling with holes for two little legs.

We'd set up a folding table, boxes of vaccines, and boxes for collecting sharps, and wait for the crowd to come.

Before long, people would start to emerge from the surrounding bush, many having walked single-track sand trails since before sun-up to get there in time. The children were transported on their mothers' backs, wrapped in *capulanas,* brightly coloured cloths used for everything from bandages to bedsheets, curtains, and tablecloths, but most notably for kid transport. Each mom or grandma (we rarely saw dads) would present the yellow vaccination card and growth chart for each of their children. Sometimes these were beat up and hard to read, but I can't remember anyone showing up without one. We would put the kids in the slings and get their weight, plot their growth on the chart, and intervene if there were signs of malnutrition. Then it was on to the vaccines: drops in the mouth for polio, a shot under the skin of the arm for BCG (a vaccination that helps prevent some of the complications of tuberculosis) and another in the thigh for tetanus, diphtheria, and pertussis.

Once we were done with the babies, we'd move on to the school. Classrooms were open on the sides with cut pole frames, palm frond roofs, and a chalkboard in the front. We would give a little lecture on nutrition, malaria, or HIV and answer the kids' questions about Canada. I would get a kick out of their disbelief, telling them about the long days of summer or how in winter the lakes got so hard you could drive a truck on them. Then the kids would line up for their booster shots. Like anywhere, some kids would cringe or cry, but most were stoic and brave. I remember laughing when one kid was so happy to get his shot that he tried to sneak back in line for a second one, thinking it would make him extra healthy. Deep in rural Africa, parents and their kids knew all too well that an infection could take a life at any time, and they were ready to do what it took to keep themselves and their families safe.

The Pfizer-BioNTech COVID-19 vaccine is kept at ultra-low temperatures prior to use. Once it is thawed, it's mixed with water in a vial that gives six doses, each drawn with a one-millilitre syringe to be injected into a patient's deltoid (shoulder) muscle. On a Saturday afternoon in mid-January 2021, Gloria Welyki was as keen as that little boy in Mozambique who wanted a second shot. She sat on the edge of her walker seat outside the common room at the LutherCare Village retirement home in Saskatoon, watching every step as we unpacked the cooler to thaw the vials of vaccine and set up our stations with Band-Aids and cotton balls and sharps containers. Gloria wanted to be first in line. She just couldn't wait to get her shot and get back to something resembling normal life. While we waited, she told me her story and why she was so excited to have the protection of the vaccine.

Gloria talked about her life with Wally, about the businesses they'd run and their eventual retirement to Emma Lake. Sadly, shortly after that lake home was lost in a fire, Wally's health went downhill as his Parkinson's disease brought dementia and depression. With Wally in long-term care and her daughters in the States, the pandemic was a lonely time for Gloria. Asked about what made her so keen for the vaccine, she spoke of seeing people again and of wanting to protect her own health. "I just wanted to live," she said. She'd lost good friends to the virus and she "wasn't ready to go." She was also alarmed by those who didn't want the vaccine. "After all of this," she wondered, "why wouldn't you want to protect yourself and others?"

The vaccine blitz at Gloria's retirement home was organized by Dr. Satchan Takaya, an infectious disease specialist whose energy and enthusiasm are as contagious as COVID. She was leading the Saskatoon vaccination campaign and had recruited doctors to come out and deliver the shots. It felt like the social event of the season, as we rushed about setting up shop and then listened to the stories of seniors and their reasons for getting immunized. Those stories, of lives lived and continuing to be lived, only served to highlight the cruelty of those who advocated against measures to stop COVID-19 because they thought the lives of elderly people weren't worth the trouble. That day we vaccinated over a hundred people, tracking down everyone we could to give them their shots. We managed to reach nearly every resident, as well as the staff on duty, those who came in on their day off, and even some who came from other homes nearby.

At the end of the day, there were a handful of doses left over and I got my shot as well. Because I was working at the Lighthouse emergency shelter and was on the roster to start working in hospital on the COVID ward, I'd been included in the first round of eligibility. At that time, eligible seniors and health care workers got a phone call from the health authority to set up a vaccination appointment. Contrary to what I would encourage others to do, when I first got that call I refused, not wanting to take what were then precious and rare doses away from others or give any impression I was jumping the line because of my political position. In the same spirit, I didn't want to see any doses wasted, wanted to encourage others to get their shots, and was happy to get my first dose that day. I rolled up my sleeve and one of the docs jabbed my right shoulder. I was more moved than I'd expected, feeling a great sense of relief. While I'd been confidently living life, sending kids to school and working in politics and medicine, the fear of catching COVID and either getting sick myself or, worse, passing it on to someone at higher risk – that fear was real. It was an incredible feeling to know that I and everyone else getting their shot finally had some protection and a reason to hope.

Medical Miracle

Thinking back to that time, it's hard to represent just how remarkable that situation was. Here we were, a year after the first case of a novel pathogen, a completely new infection, and we were distributing a safe, effective vaccine. This was truly a miracle of modern science. When we first started talking about flattening the curve to space out the infections or delay transmission until there was an effective treatment or vaccine, I was skeptical that it would be any time soon. Vaccine development is usually a long process, often taking ten to fifteen years from the initial idea to an approved vaccine.[1] Three major factors contributed to the speed of development of the COVID-19 vaccine: the decision by researchers in China to immediately sequence the genome of the newly identified coronavirus and share it and samples of the virus with scientists around the world, the coincidental emergence of mRNA vaccine technology, and Operation Warp Speed (the US government program that invested $18 billion in emergency funding for vaccine development).[2]

On December 9, 2020, exactly a year after the first cases of COVID started to emerge in Wuhan, China, the Pfizer-BioNTech COVID-19 vaccine was approved for use in Canada. Another mRNA vaccine from Moderna was approved in late December. Non-mRNA vaccines from

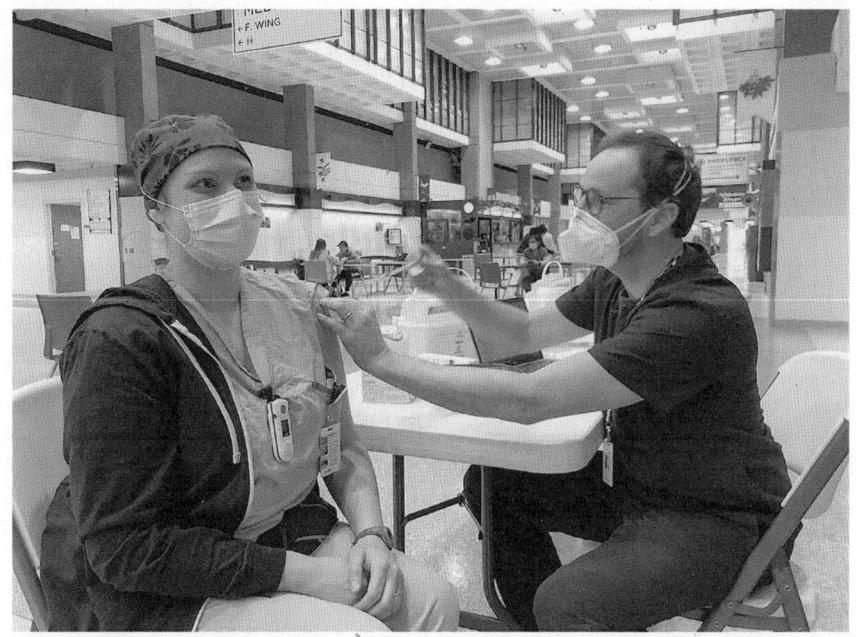

Vaccinating health care staff at Royal University Hospital
(with Katie Peters, RN). January 2022

AstraZeneca and Johnson and Johnson were approved in February and March, respectively. These vaccines would have differences in efficacy, side effects, and availability, but the fact that a year after the pandemic was declared we had four safe, effective vaccines was a scientific achievement akin to landing on the moon.

A week after that first approval, on December 15, Regina intensive care specialist Dr. Jeffrey Betcher and ER nurse Leah Sawatsky became the first people in Saskatchewan to receive a COVID-19 vaccine. In the middle of a punishing second wave, this was cause for great excitement and hope. The initial messages from the premier and health minister were sensible and encouraging. It started off well.

In those first few months, rather than the resistance to vaccination that would dominate later debates, we heard much more about those keen to get their shots. The initial rollout focused on those most at risk, with seniors over eighty, the clinically vulnerable, and health care workers receiving calls directly from the Saskatchewan Health Authority to get their appointments. After that first phase, the vaccine eligibility was rolled out by ten-year age increments, and people eagerly lined up in their cars for hours at drive-through immunization clinics when their number was called.

The SHA staff did a tremendous job with so many aspects of the pandemic response. People found themselves working longer hours than ever at their jobs or thrust into new roles of leadership. The vaccine roll-out was no exception, as the health care team used every creative means they could to reach people. There were mass immunization sites and pop-up vaccine campaigns in seniors' homes and low-income communities. I signed up for clinics at Merlis Belsher Place, the university hockey arena that had originally been designated for a field hospital. I also joined more pop-up clinics, including driving with a colleague to seniors' centres and group homes with a cooler full of vaccine, and helping immunize newcomers with the immigrant and refugee clinic set up by Mahli and her REACH colleagues. Later, Dr. Takaya and her team would transform a convention centre into a kid-friendly vaccine expo, complete with a Band-Aid buffet where kids could choose their favourite superhero or cartoon character to soothe their post-poke owies.

For me, the most exciting of these was vaccine blitz day at the Lighthouse. Knowing how high-risk the community was, Jeannie Coe and the nurse practitioner clinic team worked with Dr. Takaya to organize a drop-in immunization clinic. This most closely resembled the spirit of the mobile brigades in Mozambique – a bit chaotic but made to work through the energy of the team and the enthusiasm of those ready for their shots. The main floor dining area was set up with a reception table and six vaccination stations, and one of the shelter rooms was converted into an after-care waiting room where people could have a snack while waiting the obligatory fifteen minutes to be sure they didn't have a reaction. Nurses and doctors volunteered to spend the whole day immunizing everyone we could – residents, staff, first responders; we even went out in the alleys to invite people in. Mahli, who was there vaccinating too, said it was our best date night in a year. That might sound silly, but there's a real festival feeling to these blitzes, seeing tons of people after so little contact and with such a sense of joy and hope. People were excited but nervous, so we made jokes, asking every old man if he was sure he wasn't pregnant, gently teasing the young woman with her arms covered in tattoos about her fear of needles, making the most of the day.

There was one Lighthouse resident – I'll call him Eddie – whom I'd come to know well over the last couple of years; every time I was in clinic, he would come and see me. Sometimes he had a real medical issue, sometimes he wasn't in a good state and I'd have to ask him to come back later, but most days he was full of stories and bad jokes. He just wanted someone to talk to. When he came in on vaccine blitz day, he went to Dionne Stroo's table. Dionne lights up when she talks about the people she cares for. She has spent years building trust with people who have been hurt so much in their lives, showing she cares about them and leaving space for them to come to her when they're ready.

When she gave Eddie his vaccine, she started to cry. That said everything to me about how much the staff and care team love these people whom most of the world cannot. I asked her about this later and she told me, "I was just afraid they were all going to die, and nobody was going to care about it but us. These lives, these hard lives, are full of amazing stories. They've already been through so much, to lose them prematurely would be just so tragic." She spoke of how important the vaccine was with that group of people in particular. They had such a hard time masking and social distancing, and because of the trauma they've had with institutions, they can be scared to go to the hospital, so they often show up when they're too sick and it's too late. With that quick shot in Eddie's arm and the arms of all the others who made their way to us that day, she could see the lives saved as clear as day.

We Who Would Be First

Through most of that spring of 2021, Saskatchewan was outpacing the rest of the country in vaccine uptake. It's hard to know what drove that early adoption, but it's clear that the myriad efforts of the health care providers to organize easy access helped. Perhaps the fact that our second and third waves had been so bad helped drive people to want protection as well. Throughout the spring session, in response to every single question about ICUs being over capacity or deaths in long-term care, the government members would suggest that none of that mattered because

Saskatchewan was "leading the nation" in vaccinations. In mid-April, Health Minister Paul Merriman and chief medical health officer Dr. Saqib Shahab hosted a press conference. Merriman stated that "Saskatchewan continues to stick it to COVID faster than any other province in Canada,"[3] with over 300,000 vaccinations delivered across the province. Eighty percent of those seventy and older had their first shot by then, as did over half of those fifty and over.

Just as Saskatchewan's nation-leading first-wave response collapsed into deadly second, third, and fourth waves, the early vaccination success did not hold. In mid-May, the premier announced a "Re-Opening Roadmap" based on vaccination coverage. The idea was that if a certain percentage was reached, then public health measures were no longer needed. The plan was for some measures to be removed if 70 percent of those over forty had their first dose, a second phase of easing when we reached 70 percent of those over thirty, and then all restrictions removed when 70 percent of those over eighteen had their first shot. This was a hopeful but flawed approach.

The percentage of vaccination coverage matters, but case counts, hospitalizations, and rates of community transmission need to be taken into account as well. We also needed to remember that the percentage reflected only first doses for a vaccine that required two doses for full effect. To suggest, as the premier did, that reaching those levels would mean the end of the need for public health measures for good was wishful thinking at best and clearly reckless behaviour. Rather than promoting vaccine uptake, this approach had the opposite effect. From the moment the reopening plan was released, the implicit message to the public was "we're good now, move on."

A study from the Saskatchewan Population Health and Evaluation Research Unit (SPHERU) showed that those who had lower education levels or whose livelihoods were at greater risk were more hesitant about getting the vaccine,[4] showing the importance of both clear public communication and financial support for those in need. The degree of local threat from coronavirus also played a role, further underlining the need for reliable local information. Those who were not planning to be vaccinated were also less likely to wear masks and practise physical distancing. The removal of those measures further undermined the demand for vaccines. Study lead Dr. Nazeem Muhajarine told the CBC that "lifting the mask mandate is actually counter to getting people vaccine doses."[5] People who were hesitant about vaccination took the messaging from the premier that they didn't have to confront that discomfort.

To try to counter this, Vicki Mowat and I called for a "Last Mile Strategy" of targeted measures to reach full vaccination coverage.[6] This included removing barriers to access by returning to the model established for the highest-risk health care workers and seniors, with people receiving a call and an appointment rather than just being asked to go find it themselves. Along with booking an appointment, the callers would have been trained to explore and address questions of vaccine hesitancy and provide information on safety and efficacy. We also called for dedicated clinics in areas with low uptake and a vaccine lottery that offered a draw for cash, Roughrider tickets, bursaries, and other prizes. This was modelled on what Manitoba had done with its Vax to Win lottery, which had contributed to an increase from 68 percent with first doses in June to 85 percent in October.

Unfortunately, unlike the brief window the previous spring, the Sask Party was back in "we'll take no lessons" mode, and no added efforts to broaden vaccination coverage were made until late in the fourth wave. Starting in May, the province was eclipsed by every other part of the country, falling from first to competing day-by-day with Alberta for dead last in June and beyond. Despite those falling rates, and despite modelling showing that things were about to get a lot worse, Scott Moe and company doubled down on their planned full re-opening, calling it "a time for us to pause and be very proud of what we have achieved."[7]

As the fourth wave would very quickly prove, it was not the time to pause. However, despite the shortcomings of the province's response, there was truth in the premier's statement. Many, many people did the right thing. People got the shots for themselves, but more often the reasons I heard stemmed from concern for others. Business owners wanted to keep their customers and staff safe. Parents wanted to bring their kids to see grandparents without having to be afraid that the visit would make them sick. Health care workers wanted to be sure they wouldn't bring anything to their patients. So they stepped up, got the shot, and encouraged others to do the same.

Miracles to Come

This was great news, because the vaccines are safe and they work. The COVID vaccines have, despite the hype to the contrary, very similar safety profiles to the wide battery of vaccines that we currently employ against everything from influenza to measles. Serious adverse events following the vaccines are exceedingly rare, at about 1 in 10,000.[8] That doesn't mean they don't happen, and that they aren't real problems when they do. This is the awful calculus of public health: no intervention has zero risk; we must choose what is the least dangerous. The fact remains that the risk of becoming seriously ill from COVID is much, much higher than any risk posed by the vaccine.

And when it comes to that serious illness, even with the greater level of vaccine escape with later variants, the mRNA COVID vaccines are incredibly effective.[9] They reduce the chance of transmission and substantially reduce the likelihood of serious illness or death.[10] The C.D. Howe Institute estimates that, along with preventing billions of dollars in economic damages, COVID-19 vaccination campaigns led to a decrease in hospitalizations of 3 percent and saved 35,000 Canadian lives from January 2021 to May 2022.[11]

In a century of public health progress, vaccines have been an incredibly effective weapon against disease. They have allowed humanity to eliminate smallpox, vastly reduce the illness burden of polio, and save countless lives by preventing childhood illnesses like diphtheria, pertussis (whooping cough), chicken pox, mumps, measles, and more. There are vaccines that prevent meningitis, pneumonia, and certain kinds of cancers. The problem is, when you're winning, the enemy doesn't go away, it just becomes invisible. We have become comfortable in our success and now are at risk of losing ground. My great fear is that the rise of anti-vaccine sentiment against COVID vaccines won't stay there. We are already starting to see a drop in rates of routine vaccinations. Despite an increase in influenza infections in 2022, the number of people getting their flu shots is just over half[12] that of the previous year[13] in Saskatchewan and significantly lower all across Canada.[14] Headed into the 2022 school year, only 55 percent of Toronto students were up to date with their routine immunizations.[15] January 2023 saw a large pertussis outbreak in areas of Southern Alberta with low vaccination rates.[16] In Saskatchewan, the rate of vaccination for measles and whooping cough dropped from 81 percent in 2018 to 73 percent in 2022.[17] This is a serious problem as measles is highly contagious; you need 95 percent coverage to prevent outbreaks. Dr. Ayisha Kurji, a Saskatoon pediatrician, points out that these numbers matter: "You're actually looking at hundreds of kids who are now behind or unimmunized. And that can make a huge difference in terms of seeing some of the diseases that we have vaccinations for and shouldn't be seeing."[18]

We shouldn't assume these drops are entirely due to anti-vaccine sentiment. In fact, a 2022 National Institute on Ageing survey found that 31 percent of older Canadians reported their view of vaccination had become more positive since the beginning of the pandemic.[19] However, the disruption in schools and other parts of normal life has created barriers for parents to bring their children in for vaccines. Public health professionals have been frequently redeployed to focus on COVID, impeding the usual vaccine promotion and distribution efforts. And multiple years of public health campaigns have exhausted the appetite for public health campaigns. That said, it's hard to believe that the heightened rhetoric around the COVID vaccine won't translate into greater vaccine hesitancy for other vaccines. Seeing a moment of hope turned into a moment of fear, and the choice of some politicians to lean into the lies and endanger lives, is a tremendous disappointment. It's hard not to be discouraged as I think back to the excitement that accompanied those *brigadas* in Mozambique to wedge politics now turning people away from free, effective ways of keeping themselves and those around them safe.

There is, however, a more hopeful side to all of this. The true silver lining of these challenging years may be the prevention of diseases that take millions of lives every year. The mRNA technology used in COVID vaccines was first developed for rabies and later Ebola.[20] These are serious problems, but being diseases that plague the Global South, they have not seen the investment they should. This could be changing, with trials now underway for vaccines for some of the world's deadliest infectious diseases, including malaria and HIV.[21] There is also hope for mRNA prevention of cancers such as pancreatic cancer, colorectal cancer, and melanoma.[22] We are seeing increasing commitment to research and production of vaccines, including the establishment of Canada's first level 3 commercial vaccine development centre at the University of Saskatchewan's Vaccine and Infectious Disease Organization (VIDO).[23]

The hope is real, but so is the risk. Humanity has a stark choice: Will we learn from this experience and save countless lives by progressing in both our scientific understanding and our distribution of the elements of good health? Or will we regress, becoming more isolated, suspicious of the very things that can save us? The power to choose a healthier future is in our hands.

Variants of Concern

One morning in mid-April 2021, I visited my dad, Wally Meili, in the ICU at Regina General Hospital. He was intubated, recovering from brain surgery. I learned from the nurses on the unit that there were so many seriously ill COVID patients in the unit that they were having to double-bunk, putting two patients in rooms designed for one. One nurse said to me, "It's like a nightmare we can't wake up from." I then drove straight from the hospital to the legislature to ask the premier about it during question period. The collision of my personal, medical, and political lives left me reeling.

Regina was under siege that spring. Case counts had soared as the Alpha variant hit the city hard. Travel was officially discouraged to and from the city. The legislature had convened for a modified sitting – five days a week over six weeks instead of the usual four days a week spread over the entire spring – and the MLAs had to stay in the city the entire time. This was hard on all of the out-of-town MLAs, but especially those with young kids. I know many greater sacrifices were made through the pandemic, and that parents often had to be away from their families for long stretches, but that was the hardest time for me. I talked to my boys via FaceTime, and we sent each other letters and little gifts, but I could tell it was hard on them for us to be so far apart.

And, although we were back in the legislature in person, we were apart there as well. Each desk had a sheet of Plexiglas in front of it and only half of the MLAs were allowed in the chamber at a time. We held our caucus meetings via Zoom. To facilitate spacing, members from the government side were seated next to the opposition. This also facilitated some of their louder members shouting in my ear when I would try to ask the premier questions.

Under Pressure

A week after we started the session, I got a call from my mom, Lea. Dad hadn't come home from the office the night before. Before taking over the family farm from my grandfather, Walter, he had sold houses in Moose Jaw, and when he retired from the farm he'd returned to real estate. Fifty years later, he still loved meeting people and getting them started in a new home or business. Something of a workaholic, he hadn't slowed down at all, so a late night at work was nothing strange. But then his colleague found him lying on the floor of his office, unconscious, at five in the morning. At the Moose Jaw hospital, a CT scan of his head showed that he'd had a hemorrhagic stroke: one of the blood vessels in his brain had burst, causing a major bleed. A repeat scan in Regina showed the bleed had worsened and he would need emergency life-saving surgery.

We had no idea whether he would survive the surgery or the weeks to follow, let alone whether he would walk or speak again. He was in the ICU for six days, hospital for six weeks, and rehab in Moose Jaw for two months. His recovery has been incredible in many ways. His doctors said that most people his age would never walk again, but Wally wasn't most people his age. At seventy-four he was in better shape than most fifty-year-olds. That meant he was more likely to recover, but also that the losses in function were more deeply felt.

At fifteen years of age, Wally started doing fifteen push-ups every morning. He increased that by one every birthday. At seventy he started doing two sets of fifty, because he'd decided he should live to be a hundred. He'd be finished his exercises and an hour or two of work before anyone else in the house woke up. Inherent in that was a bit of latent disappointment in everyone around him who couldn't keep up. Now it's the opposite. He has learned to walk again and can handle the stairs slowly. His long-term memory and memory for people is great. But he sleeps most of the day and gets grouchy if you try to get him moving.

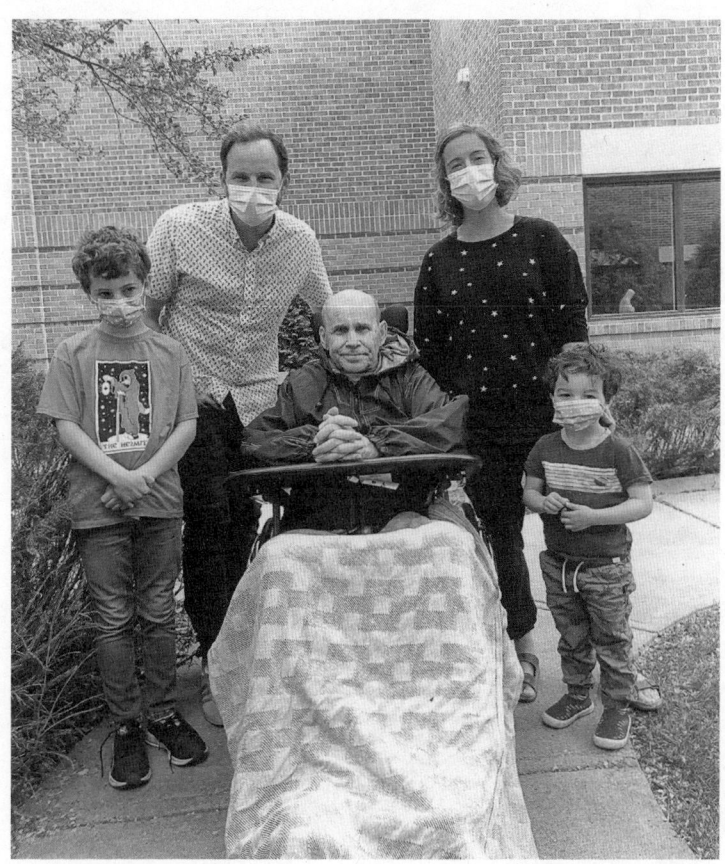

Visiting my dad, Wally, in Moose Jaw after his stroke
with my wife Mahli, Abe, and Gus. May 2021

It's one of the hardest things to accept about being human: how much of who we are is stored in the jelly-like grey matter in our skulls, and how a minor change in that physical structure can change our supposedly immutable character and self. It's hard for the person who changes, and even harder for those they love.

Mom stayed with me at my Regina apartment that entire session, walking every day to see Wally at the hospital. We were grateful even that was allowed, as many people weren't getting any visits, though also aware that privilege was a function of how seriously ill he was. We would have gladly had him too well to visit! Lea is as hard-working as Dad, though she was never dialled up quite as high, preferring to sleep in until the ungodly hour of 8:00 a.m. before diving into the day. She is one of the most patient and kindest people I've ever met, qualities that made her an excellent nurse and later administrator of a seniors' home in Moose Jaw. It's also meant that, as exhausting as it has been to accompany Wally through his recovery and adapt to the changes in his personality, there is no one better suited to be by his side.

When you're an MLA, you don't enter the legislative chambers by the main door. That's for the speaker, the lieutenant governor, and special guests on special occasions. The members enter by side doors, giving a bow in the direction of the speaker's chair if the house is in session. Across a hallway from the side doors are the members' lounges, one for the government, the other for the opposition. One day, after question period, we were getting ready for scrums and my chief of staff, Sally Housser, asked me if I was okay. And as with Dr. Shahab, that was the question I wasn't ready for. I choked back the tears and told her no, I wasn't okay. And I did something I never do – I took the next day off and stayed away, visiting my dad in ICU but not able to face the legislature.

What had particularly struck me, I explained to Sally, was the realization that Dad had received his COVID-19 vaccine just a few days before his stroke. We would eventually learn that Wally had a rare cancer called amyloidosis that had destroyed one of the proteins in his blood needed for clotting to happen. That's why his brain started to bleed; it had nothing to do with the vaccine. But at that moment, the thought that the vaccine I was so proudly and vigorously promoting might have hurt my own family was an enormously heavy thing to imagine. The statistics are right, the likelihood of a bad outcome is hundreds of times greater from the virus than the vaccine. But if someone you love dies in a plane crash, the fact that it was far safer statistically than driving in a car is not at all comforting. And yet that's the position that everyone promoting the best possible response with the information we had at the time was in. It wasn't do no harm, take no risk; it was do the least harm.

I was recently at a celebration of life for Mary and Dr. C. Stuart Houston. Dr. Houston was an eminent radiologist, ornithologist, and author from Saskatoon. He passed away in July 2021, a couple of years after his wife, Mary. Their son Stan spoke of how diminished Stuart's final months were as he lost the ability to connect with his community as he had so vigorously done throughout his life. Stan is an infectious disease physician, and he spoke of the paradox of knowing how necessary the public health measures were, of fully supporting them, and also knowing that the damage they caused was real. These are difficult decisions, the sacrifices are real, but you still have to make the right choices.

It's worth noting that we saw Scott Moe show emotion a couple of times during those first two years of the pandemic.[1] In the spring of 2021, he teared up in the legislature, and that emotion was real. What struck me was that what moved him was having to isolate seniors from their families. He later described this and having young people unable to participate in things like hockey or school dances as his great regrets.[2] These are legitimate things to be sorry about, if not necessarily sorry for. What was striking to me is that he has appeared to be more concerned with the knock-on effects of when he did the right thing than the effects of when he failed to. Early on, there were messages of condolences in the press briefings, but as the death count climbed, the premier and health minister stopped mentioning lives lost and stopped expressing concern and care for the families of those in the ICU. It was a notable shift and one that was hard to understand. Had they developed a blind spot to this suffering, having decided it was no longer their problem? Or did they think that by acknowledging the deaths they were admitting their failures? Perhaps, but instead of avoiding that scrutiny, they gave the strong impression that they cared more about those inconvenienced in their lives than those who lost them entirely.

That seeming indifference extended to the double-bunked Regina ICU. After visiting the Regina ICU, I contacted Dr. Jeff Betcher, the department head, to learn more about what was happening. He told me how overwhelmed they were in the unit, with people dying daily and more sick patients every day to replace them. He wanted to show me how serious things were, and invited me to tour the unit and said he would welcome the premier as well. I asked the premier to join me in touring the ICU and he refused.[3] His excuse was that this wasn't fair as families couldn't visit. For one, that wasn't the case. I knew from experience with my dad that the ICU was the one place where families were allowed. Instead, even when Dr. Betcher urged him to visit through media interviews,[4] Moe wouldn't go, and the Saskatchewan Health Authority stepped in to stop me from visiting as well. Given there was no legitimate objection to the premier seeing the unit, I can only conclude that he didn't want to be seen anywhere near the site of a disaster he had a hand in creating.

Losing the Race

Perhaps what is most sad about the level of death and disease we saw that spring in Regina was how completely predictable and preventable it was. The failure to get ahead of the second wave led to much longer business restrictions than a circuit breaker would have. The clearest demonstration of that missed opportunity is the contrast with the experience in Atlantic Canada.

From the beginning, the Atlantic provinces of Nova Scotia, Newfoundland and Labrador, New Brunswick, and Prince Edward Island took COVID more seriously than the rest of Canada. Rather than wanting to be the first, they strove to be the best. This included a slower reopening in the summer of 2020 and the establishment of the Atlantic Bubble, which enforced a strict quarantine for out-of-province travellers but allowed free travel between the four provinces. They also invested heavily in test-trace-isolate capacity to get on top of any stray cases. Case numbers and mortality were lower under Atlantic Canada's containment model than in the six provinces to their west that pursued a reactive "mitigation" strategy.[5] Rather than prolonged and painful, the second and third waves in the East were short and sharp. This also allowed Atlantic Canadians to live much more normal lives, with fewer restrictions required because they were able to keep their case counts low.

At the end of April 2021, Nova Scotia introduced a circuit breaker lockdown in response to an increase in cases. These measures were introduced when cases were at a rate of fifteen per hundred thousand, in contrast to the non-Atlantic provinces, which waited until rates were nearly ten times that high.[6] In Saskatchewan, rather than our having time to recover, the third wave arrived while we were still dealing with the second. This constructive interference increased both the health and

Third Wave

economic damage. By contrast, the Atlantic provinces saw their employment rates bounce back more quickly,[7] giving the lie to the idea that we had to sacrifice lives for livelihoods. For example, traffic in bars and restaurants declined by 21 percent in the Atlantic provinces in 2021, 42 percent in the provinces that said they were keeping things open.[8] Nova Scotia premier Iain Rankin made the case for this approach, saying that "the best economic policy is a strong public health policy."[9] As of October 2022, each of the Atlantic provinces had posted death rates less than half that of Saskatchewan, and for Prince Edward Island, New Brunswick, and Nova Scotia, population growth rates more than double.[10]

An academic study on the differences in provincial and territorial responses described the situation clearly: "The Atlantic provinces of New Brunswick, Nova Scotia, Prince Edward Island and Newfoundland and Labrador have experienced more freedoms and 'normality' over the course of the COVID-19 pandemic than the larger more populous central and western provinces."[11] This was one of a number of papers published in the first year of the pandemic that demonstrated the superiority of this approach for all of the factors provincial leaders cited as important: health system protection, economic recovery, and return to normal life.[12] Sadly, just as with the failure to protect seniors' homes despite having seen what happened in Quebec and Ontario, Saskatchewan and other governments ignored the Atlantic success.

In Saskatchewan, the opposite approach meant that gathering limits and other restrictions introduced reluctantly and half-heartedly in the fall had to be continued into the spring. By failing to act quickly and decisively, the Moe government had prolonged both the outbreaks and the measures needed to address them. The premier started to show his impatience with this situation in February 2021, accusing those who were calling for a more effective response of acting from privilege when he said that "it's easy for some to stand up and say, 'We need to lock everything down,' when they have the opportunity to work from home."[13] Only, the loudest voices for more measures weren't some ill-defined laptop class. His comments were a slap in the face to the doctors and nurses speaking up from the frontlines. These were the people who couldn't work from home, people whose professions put them at the greatest risk, a risk made worse by his government's choices. A couple of days later, he would soften those remarks, saying, "We're not going to just open this up. That would be entirely disrespectful to those folks that are going to work every day, are on the frontlines treating patients that may or may not have COVID." But very shortly after he would do exactly that.

In late February, chief medical health officer Dr. Saqib Shahab described the situation as a race between the vaccine and the variants as cases of the newly identified B.1.1.7 or Alpha variant were identified in Regina.[14] On March 4, in one of the biweekly Physician Town Hall webinars hosted by the Saskatchewan Health Authority, Saskatchewan doctors were presented with slides showing Saskatchewan leading the country in cases and deaths, and informed of the urgency posed by increased variants of concern in the province.[15] They were told that case rate and rate of transmission had not yet met the SHA's goals and that despite a "small but vocal minority" calling for "relaxing" measures, existing restrictions needed to stay in place until at least March 19. Despite this information, which, if available to the province's physicians, was surely on the desk of the premier, Scott Moe chose to reduce restrictions on March 9, increasing gathering limits and household bubbles. Epidemiologist Nazeem Muhajarine told the media: "I fear that this could actually touch off a third wave, because the variants are so difficult to control ... Lifting restrictions at the same time [as variants of concern are emerging], it's a recipe for disaster."[16]

Modelling shared at the next doctors' town hall showed a massive increase in ICU admissions without new measures. Not long after, Dr. Shahab would question the government's approach, writing to colleagues in the SHA that "the current strategy is not enough. Any protection the vaccine provides currently will fail if case numbers are allowed to go too high as they are going now."[17] This exchange reveals just how much the government was calling the shots, with public health leadership having to carry water for their decisions and the public paying the price.

Two weeks after the premier lifted restrictions, Regina had the highest proportion of variants of concern anywhere in Canada. The province prohibited private gatherings in Regina, closed indoor dining and non-essential indoor facilities, and erected a huge sign on the highway advising against travel in and out of the provincial capital. Instead of short-term restrictions to get ahead of the rising waves, we were six months into a slow-motion lockdown that fell far short of protecting lives or livelihoods. This is the lesson that seems so hard for governments, especially conservative governments, to learn. When you try to save money by sacrificing people's lives, you lose both. When you act too slowly, not only is it callous disregard for the loss of human life to immediate illness, it undermines the economic recovery necessary for long-term health. And for those who must work, whose jobs are too essential to stay home, the risk is even greater.

Workers at Risk

"Dr. Shaw, I'm alive." Nearly two weeks after Dianne Desjarlais Cardinal had shared the story of her son Matthew's admission to the ICU on social media, Matthew replied with this message to a tweet from chief medical officer Dr. Susan Shaw, who had shared his story and encouraged Matthew in his recovery.[18] Matty Cardinal was thirty-four, and the severity of his illness brought home how the virus had changed, affecting younger people still ineligible for vaccine protection.

On St. Patrick's Day, Matty's chest felt heavy as the converted access bus drove him to the COVID-19 testing centre in Regina. He'd started feeling tired a couple of days earlier, then developed a headache, fever, and nosebleed. He called in sick to the restaurant where he was working as a server and where he most likely caught COVID-19. He'd been extremely careful, always masking and sanitizing, and being very diligent about requiring clients to register their names for contact tracing. He believes a customer who used a fake name brought the virus into the restaurant.

On the second day, he lost his sense of smell and started to cough. His Fitbit told him he needed to stop exercising, even though he was lying in bed, his sheets soaked with sweat. When he took the SHA bus in for testing, the driver opened the windows and the testing staff rushed him through, as they could all see he was quite sick. The test came back positive on a Saturday. On the Monday he was feeling exhausted and lethargic. He tried to take a hot shower to revive himself, and instead he found himself gasping for breath and feeling like he was going to die.

He was able to call 911 and the ambulance took him to the emergency room at the Regina General Hospital, where they started him on oxygen. The ER doc told him that he was in bad shape, that they would try their best, but it didn't look good.

He continued to get worse over the following days, feeling like he was slowly dying as he required more and more oxygen. The staff asked him if he wanted to be resuscitated. When he told them he wanted to live, he was transferred to the ICU. He tried to call some friends and family, but no one was answering their phones, so he posted a message on Facebook, essentially saying goodbye. Shortly afterward he was surrounded by the intensive care team and he asked them to "please try to save my life" just before he was intubated. Six days later they were able to remove the breathing tube, and that's when he sent his message to Dr. Shaw, sending relief to so many who were watching for news of his recovery.

Ten days later, with the aid of oxygen and a walker, he was able to climb stairs and dress himself well enough to be sent home. Before he was even discharged, he was already speaking out to try to protect others who were at risk of the same outcome. He spoke with *Saskatoon StarPhoenix* reporter Zak Vescera, describing the young frontline workers he'd seen in the ICU, and called for delivery drivers, grocery store workers, and first responders to be vaccinated.[19] His advocacy helped change the Saskatchewan vaccine schedule as the province altered it to include fire, police, and more frontline workers in mid-April.[20]

Out of hospital, he continued to speak out as an advocate for smart policy to prevent COVID transmission, all while trying to recover from his traumatic brush with death. He pushed himself to walk around Wascana Park only a few days after leaving hospital. It took him three-and-a-half hours and lots of breaks on his walker to complete the four-kilometre loop, but he made it. By continuing those walks he was able to get off oxygen and ditch the walker in two weeks and return to work shortly after.

Matty has cooked, served, and managed in many restaurants. He would like to open a restaurant of his own someday. He wants to start with a food truck and build up the reputation and collateral to start a multicultural fusion restaurant in Regina. He has big dreams, but he also recognizes that it isn't going to be easy. He describes himself as operating at 90 percent of what he was before COVID. He's trying to be grateful, knowing he's lucky to be here at all, but it's not always easy. The day we met to talk about his experience, he had stood lost in a nearby grocery store for a few minutes before remembering where he was going. These episodes of brain fog are frequent, and he is still tired and short of breath. He now has a chronic lung condition called bronchitis obliterans organizing pneumonia and has to take puffers and oral steroids to keep it under control. Every time he gets sick, including when he caught the Omicron variant of COVID, he's knocked out for days. And, as the detail and emotion with which he tells his story show, he's been mentally traumatized as well. He still wakes with dreams of being unable to breathe and struggles with anxiety and hopelessness. One of the ways he's trying to use his experience for the good is by working with university researchers on studies related to long COVID and on the experience of the pandemic in Saskatchewan.

Matty's experience reminds us of two important things. One is that we don't understand the long-term effects of COVID-19. Long COVID, while increasingly understood as the persistence of physical symptoms like fatigue, shortness of breath, and cough, and psychological symptoms such as confusion, depression, and post-traumatic stress disorder, is still a mystery. When we are discussing the cost of prevention, we need to remember that the total cost of this disease may be far more than the immediate infection.

Second, his story reminds us of the precariousness of people's jobs. While everyone's life was disrupted by COVID, exactly how varied greatly based on the type of work people did. Some people were able to keep doing their jobs from home, working online and meeting co-workers by phone and Zoom. Some saw their jobs disappear overnight and were reliant on Employment Insurance or CERB. Others had to be on-site, their work declared essential. This latter group ranged from grocery store clerks and gas station attendants to people employed in industries like construction and mining, to health care workers on the frontlines of the COVID response.

COVID clearly revealed how much people's incomes were at the mercy of illness. Workers sick from or exposed to COVID had to either go in to work and take the risk of getting sicker or passing the virus on to others or else miss out on pay they couldn't afford to lose. Several jurisdictions introduced temporary sick leave during the pandemic, and British Columbia now has a permanent policy of five paid sick days per employee. A study in the United States showed that cities with paid sick leave had a 17 percent higher vaccination rate than those without.[21] For its part, the Government of Saskatchewan introduced a three-hour leave for people getting their vaccines but did not extend that program to parents taking their children for vaccines.[22]

Ali Syed worked at the power station at Boundary Dam. He is believed to have caught COVID from a SaskPower co-worker while carpooling to the job. In April 2021, his wife delivered their third child by C-section while admitted to hospital with COVID. Shortly after, Ali died in the ICU at the same hospital.[23] This unbelievably tragic story further highlighted the need for people who are sick to stay home and keep themselves and those around them safe. Recognizing it is those with the least job security that tend to have the least coverage, NDP labour critic Jennifer Bowes introduced legislation to have ten days of paid sick leave per year for all Saskatchewan employees. The Sask Party voted down the bill, leaving more than half of Saskatchewan workers without any sick leave coverage.

Canadian wages have not been keeping up with the cost of living for many years. The Fight for $15 campaign started in the United States as a labour movement effort to increase the federal minimum wage to $15 per hour.[24] That movement spread to Canada, and in 2018 Alberta became the first province to make its minimum wage $15. Saskatchewan has been in a race to the bottom with New Brunswick for the lowest minimum wage for the better part of a decade, leaving people working full-time jobs living below the poverty line.[25] Pushed by the rising cost of living and growing labour shortages, the Sask Party finally agreed to increase the minimum wage to $13 an hour in October 2022 and continue increasing it to $15 in 2024. This is a victory for advocates of increasing wages, but still leaves Saskatchewan with the lowest minimum wage in the country, and the cost of living continues to rise. A living wage in Saskatchewan was calculated at $16.23 in Regina and $16.89 in Saskatoon in 2021, and that number has surely risen with recent inflation.[26]

If we want working people to thrive instead of just barely survive, we have to be shooting beyond the bare minimum for wages and working conditions that allow people to meet their basic needs. Working people deserve to earn a living wage. Workers like Matty have done so much of the heavy lifting these last three years, just as they do every other year. First responders, delivery drivers, servers, grocery clerks – they've been taking great risks with little reward. Much was made of thanking these workers, especially in the early days of the pandemic. Those thanks ring hollow as we appear to be on a path to once again accept exploitation and the resultant suffering as the unavoidable cost of doing business. When people earn good wages, their lives and the lives of those around them improve. They spend more locally and build up the economy. If we want to grow our province and our country, if we want the people who make this place their home to live great lives, then making sure people have jobs that are well-paying, secure, and safe is a terrific place to start.

Fourth Wave

They considered themselves free
and no one will ever be free as long as there is
plague, pestilence and famine.

– Albert Camus, *The Plague*

Total cases in Canada	380,000
Total cases in Saskatchewan	56,368
Deaths from COVID in Canada	3,329
Deaths from COVID in Saskatchewan	693

Provincial Public Health Measures

July 11, 2021	Saskatchewan is first province in Canada to lift all public health orders
September 10, 2021	Mandatory ten-day self-isolation after a positive test result re-introduced
September 17, 2021	Province-wide public mask mandate reinstated
October 1, 2021	Proof-of-vaccination or negative test required to access many public spaces

Best Summer Ever

On July 7, 2021, a little over a year into the pandemic, Scott Moe held his last regular public briefing with Dr. Saqib Shahab, broadcast from the Radio Room at the legislature. We had become accustomed to these events, with the premier and the chief medical health officer seated six feet apart at a long oak desk framed by three Canadian flags and three Saskatchewan flags. This was where they had delivered updates on case trends, public health measures, and vaccine updates. It was also nearly the only place where journalists could ask direct questions, albeit in a much more controlled fashion than a scrum in the rotunda of the legislature.

At the end of the briefing, Moe referenced having said, in March 2020, that he looked forward to the day he could shake Dr. Shahab's hand.[1] He noted that they were both at least two weeks past their second doses and hoped to take that opportunity to safely shake his hand and "thank you properly for the effort that you have made on behalf of all Saskatchewan residents." The two men shook hands and the press conference ended. It was a nice moment, and the recognition of Dr. Shahab's sacrifice and dedication was well deserved.

Unfortunately, the symbolism of that handshake went beyond acknowledging Dr. Shahab's leadership. In the same briefing, Moe declared that, based on first doses of vaccines, we had reached the end of his Re-Opening Roadmap, and all public health restrictions would end on July 11. This included masking mandates, any gathering restrictions, and even the requirement to self-isolate when testing positive for COVID-19. The premier nodded to the growing rhetoric that framed any public health measures as an assault on individual freedoms, saying that the time when the province would use government intervention to control COVID was over. He denied the presence of a "mission accomplished" banner behind him, referencing President George W. Bush's failed declaration of victory in the second US war in Iraq. The fact that he felt the need to mention this underlined the disconnect between these words and the effect of the overall message. Whether one saw this as premature or overdue, it was impossible not to see a declaration of victory. What was intended as a tribute – to Dr. Shahab and all those who had worked hard to protect the public from the pandemic – ultimately came across as a dismissal. The implicit message was that the worst was over, people could stop worrying, stop masking, stop social distancing, and move on. It was a handshake that would turn to tears.

Ignoring the Signs, Again

The worst was not over; it was yet to come. Two months earlier, federal minister of health Patty Hajdu said that "more people need to be vaccinated before we can ease restrictions."[2] This was accompanied by advice that urged caution, including keeping indoor masking until 75 percent of the eligible population had received their second dose. Moe's response was to tweet that "we won't be having a Trudeau summer here. We're going to have a great Saskatchewan summer,"[3] echoing his pre-election tweet that there would be no second wave. A few days later, Jason Kenney announced that Alberta was going to have the "Best Summer Ever,"[4] and in July posted a photo of himself shaking hands with Moe to congratulate him on kicking off a "#GreatSKSummer."[5] That "Great Saskatchewan Summer" would create the conditions for what Dr. Shahab would refer to as a "fall and winter of misery."[6]

Sending this message, as Moe had with his election eve "no more lockdowns" promise, would have been terribly irresponsible had it simply been based on conjecture. Things were changing so fast and previous declarations of an imminent end had proven so wrong that any statement about the future behaviour of the virus or risk to the public should have been qualified. Whatever their political or personal motivations, leaders need to stop giving people the false hope of simple, short-term endings. It makes it harder to motivate people to respond to future outbreaks and discourages them from taking preventive actions. As public health specialist Dr. Cory Neudorf pointed out, "by removing all the restrictions, you also remove any incentive for people who are hesitant to come forward for immunization, because you haven't set a higher bar to move to the next level of removing restrictions."[7]

Even in the face of a very promising outlook, the prudent thing to say is that things look good right now but we will have to re-evaluate should the situation change. That's if things look good. If there are signs of trouble on the horizon, one would clearly be even more cautious. Neil Sasakamoose told reporters: "Their messaging in July and August, it was the most careless messaging you could do. It was to say, 'Everyone go back to where you were.'"[8] It turns out "careless" is a generous characterization of the messaging on the day of the handshake.

A presentation titled "Risk of Fall Surge" had been prepared on June 15, just three weeks earlier, by the province's COVID modelling team.[9] The projections were based on the emerging Delta variant, the premier's plan of removing all public health measures on July 11, and the 70 percent vaccination rate underlying that decision. What it showed was alarming. The modelling projected a major surge in cases and ICU admissions into the fall of 2021. The prospect of overflowing ICUs meant that the very nightmare scenario of ethical triage – the term the experts used for putting physicians and health care administrators in the impossible position of deciding who would get care and who would be refused, of deciding who would live and who would die – had been placed on the desk of the premier. His response was to take the summer off – it would be forty-eight days, an entire Saskatchewan summer, before there was another public briefing – and encourage everyone else to do the same. Far from any sort of suppression strategy, even the idea of mitigating the impact on health care, of flattening the curve, had been tossed out with last week's three-ply masks.

The modelling proved to be, in the words of Deputy Chief Medical Health Officer, Pandemic Dr. John Froh, "remarkably accurate." For example, seventy-five ICU admissions were projected by mid-October.

When the modelling was revealed in a Physician Town Hall meeting on October 21, the actual number was seventy-eight.[10] That is notable for the accuracy, but also the timing. At that point in October, Saskatchewan was leading the country in cases, deaths, and ICU admissions per capita. We were already sending patients to Ontario ICUs because Saskatchewan hospitals simply couldn't handle the surge. Froh described how, as limits of capacity were approached and exceeded, "ethical choices about who receives [an] appropriate level of critical care and who receives substandard care are already occurring."[11] In other words, patients were at increased risk of harm and death, not only from the virus but also from the inability of the health care system to provide them with appropriate care, regardless of the illness that brought them to hospital.

The fact that doctors and the public were made aware of this modelling only in October is truly shocking, truly unprecedented, in a time where the words "shocking" and "unprecedented" had lost their meaning. There is no single moment that is more clearly a deadly abdication of responsibility, no more obvious example of political malpractice on a fatal scale. The premier wanted a good-news summer. He wanted to trash the prime minister. He wanted to go to Rider games without a mask and chum around with Jason Kenney at the Calgary Stampede. He seemed perfectly comfortable running the risk of things getting much, much worse, which is exactly what happened. It's hard to imagine how someone could so deliberately ignore the signs that were right in front of him, so blatantly choose political expediency over the public good.

There are larger issues at play than the personalities of the day, than the choices of Premier Moe and his health minister, Paul Merriman. At the same time, I couldn't completely ignore their actions or the anger they evoked. Looking at reliable scientific evidence that shows the course you're on will result in hundreds of deaths, devastate the health care system, and failing to change course is beyond incompetence. The lives of the people you are elected to represent should always be the highest priority and primary consideration.

As the fourth wave built at the end of summer and into the fall, people were calling on the opposition to do something. There was this sense that we should be able to appeal the mismanagement to some higher level, to call on the lieutenant governor to intervene or demand an emergency confidence vote. That's understandable – it seems like there ought to be some kind of release valve when a government is making terrible choices. There is no such mechanism, no immediate override of the representatives chosen by the people, and it's very hard to imagine one that wouldn't be abused. We could call for resignations – which we did – but beyond taking the case for change to the public in hopes the government would feel the pressure and act, the options for the opposition are limited.[12]

Whether it's a virtue or not depends on the moment, but I don't get mad easily. During the fourth wave, however, I was angry. Former federal NDP leader Ed Broadbent once told me that opposition is toxic to the soul. Perhaps this is what he meant. Seeing everything in the worst possible light because it's your job to point out problems skews your vision at the best of times. Being unrelentingly negative, even when that is what the job requires at a moment of extreme government failure, is exhausting. It is unbelievably frustrating to stand by and watch as people are dying and see no shame, let alone any course correction. At the end of August, this frustration boiled over in a scrum outside my MLA office in Saskatoon, where I referred to Scott Moe and Paul Merriman as "stupid, irresponsible men."[13] That's not an inaccurate description of their actions, but it's not particularly helpful. If anything, it likely caused them to dig their heels in more. On the other hand, polite and constructive criticism wasn't changing anything either. The only tool available was to channel the frustration of the people who were hurting.

That is not to say that all the measures of spring 2021 needed to stay through the summer. One of the ways to prevent COVID fatigue is to take advantage of natural windows to give people a summer break. In that June modelling, there was another projection, a line that represented vaccination of 85 percent of the eligible population and a much milder fall ICU surge as a result. How many more Saskatchewan people would be alive, how many fewer people would be waiting months more in pain for essential surgeries, had the message been different that day? What if, instead of a dramatic farewell handshake, the premier had shown people the modelling of what was to come? What if he had used that danger on the horizon to promote a "last mile" vaccination plan through the summer window, and readied people for the possibility of new public health restrictions instead of signalling it was all in the past?

We'll never know for sure, but we do know that public health experts were urging exactly that approach. Through July and August, medical officers of health in Saskatchewan worked behind the scenes to urge the government to take the modelling seriously. They got nowhere. That frustration finally boiled over in an unheard-of display of independence from a group of public employees that is traditionally reticent to diverge from public policy. Led by Dr. Neudorf, the group penned a letter at the end of August describing how rising rates of transmission of the Delta variant were already overwhelming the ability to do testing and contact tracing, and the imminent risk of overwhelming hospitals as well.[14] They called on the province to act quickly by changing the "live with COVID" messaging that was undermining the seriousness of the pending fourth wave. They also called for mandatory vaccination for health care workers and provincial and municipal employees, proof of vaccination for restaurants, bars, and other social events, and the return of mask mandates.

The premier responded to the letter by saying that, except for mandatory vaccines for some health care workers, he would not be taking the advice of these public health experts. He called the idea of proof of vaccination, something that was already in place in British Columbia and Manitoba, "heavy-handed" and said that "it won't be the government that comes out and forces such a policy."[15] Once again, presupposing what measures would be considered and vowing not to take certain steps led to a delay even he would be forced to acknowledge was a failure, though he would downplay this by saying he "potentially" should have acted "a week, possibly ten days earlier."[16]

Inmates and Outbreaks

While the fourth wave of the most visible public health emergency was building, the province's more silent epidemic continued to claim a growing number of lives. One of those lives was Cory Charles Cardinal, a well-known poet and prison reform advocate. He spoke openly about his struggles with addiction and with HIV and hepatitis C, and fought for harm reduction and the rights of those living with HIV/AIDS. He had developed relationships with reporters in Saskatoon who turned to him as a source for what was really happening in corrections and in the inner city. Cory died alone in the window well of an apartment building in downtown Saskatoon that summer, just two months after being released from prison.

Two summers earlier, I received a surprising email from the Pro Bono Law group in Regina:

My name is Cory Charles Cardinal, and I am currently remanded at the Saskatoon Provincial Correctional Center. My brother recently died on Monday. I had applied for a temporary absence to attend my brother's funeral in Prince Albert today. I was denied by corrections staff the ability to attend my brother's funeral. When questioning the corrections staff as to the reasons why I was not able to attend the funeral, I was labelled as belligerent and was taken off of my unit to the holding cells.

You may have heard about segregation in jails, but in Saskatoon Provincial there is a worse place than segregation, the holding cells, which is referred to as "The Hole". I am currently in The Hole and am relaying my message through my lawyer to the outside world. There are six inmates being held in The Hole. We are denied our one hour of exercise, a daily shower and have no access to any books. We are double bunked in our cells. We are forced to wear security-type dresses, called baby dolls. The baby dolls are not washed from the previous inmate. We are not allowed to wear shirts, or shoes. The conditions are disgusting and severely inhumane. Ants crawl on the floor, where mice are seen frequently. There is one inmate who has been down here for seven days without exercise time, a daily shower, or a book to read. I am officially protesting the conditions of The Hole by a hunger strike. I will not eat until Ryan Meili or [Opposition Justice Critic] Nicole Sarauer attend Saskatoon Provincial Correctional Centre to see the conditions.

A hunger strike is a drastic measure, and the treatment he was identifying very worrisome. It's also quite difficult to get into a Saskatchewan correctional facility to visit a prisoner. I was able to get in touch with

Cory by phone and convince him to start eating again. A few days later I drove out to the Saskatoon provincial jail, where I was taken through security and brought into a small meeting room. Cory was escorted in by a guard, sat down, and immediately started to tell me about life in jail. We had met a few times when I was working in inner-city Saskatoon, including at the annual AIDS Walk fundraiser, where he shared powerful spoken-word poetry about his experiences with addiction and HIV. I'd been impressed by his passion for improving the community and his openness about his own struggles and experiences. He told me some of his story, including an honest account of the addictions-related drug and property crimes that had landed him in jail again.

Along with being totally open about his own flaws, Cory didn't leave his activism on the outside. He started a group called Inmates for Humane Conditions, and spoke out about overcrowding, mistreatment of prisoners, and the lack of supports for people to get help and improve their lives before being returned to society. He presented me with a notebook with the logo of his group hand-drawn on the cover. Inside are the testimonies of inmates written in their own hand. They describe being denied basic dental or medical care, including receiving prescribed medications or treatment for tuberculosis. They complain of the lack of basic hygiene, with dirty cells and bathrooms, and of going ten days or more without a toothbrush or a shower. And they remark with insight on the problem of locking people up with no opportunity to go through rehabilitation or advance their education, leaving them stuck in the cycle of addictions, poverty, and crime.

Cory was still in jail for the first year of the pandemic. COVID-19 loves "congregate living" situations: places where people live in close quarters. Prisons are classic sites of added risk for infectious diseases like tuberculosis. Poor ventilation, crowded conditions, and underlying health problems leave inmate populations extremely vulnerable to outbreaks. That should be enough for governments to care; whatever their crimes, these are human beings in the care of the state. Even in the absence of such a humane viewpoint, the risk to the health care system if large outbreaks send prisoners to hospital should be reason enough to make sure the virus doesn't run wild through incarcerated populations.

The World Health Organization joined other United Nations agencies in March 2020 in calling on governments to decrease the risk of spread in jails by releasing those who could "be released without compromising public safety."[17] Early in the pandemic, a group of public defenders and legal experts identified the long-standing overcrowding of Saskatchewan correctional facilities as a risk, saying that "it is not a question of whether the virus will spread through the prisons, it is a question of how quickly," and calling for targeted early release and probation of low-risk offenders.[18] The government declined.

When the outbreaks started in earnest in Saskatchewan corrections facilities in the second wave, there were not enough spaces to house positive inmates away from those not yet infected. There were dozens of cases in Regina and Prince Albert and over a hundred guards and prisoners tested positive in Saskatoon.[19] The province doubled down on refusing to seek alternatives. Minister of Corrections and Policing Christine Tell accused advocates of seeing COVID-19 as a "get out of jail free card" and refused to investigate how the outbreaks happened.[20]

Cory spoke out about the dangers of COVID-19 to inmates at the Saskatoon Provincial Correctional Centre and the stress they were under, knowing there were many older inmates and people with underlying illnesses that put them at higher risk, all living in crowded conditions with inadequate sanitation. In a February 2021 interview, he described how, just before an outbreak was declared in his unit, "fear and distrust was rampant. Every cough was met with suspicion. There is a code that inmates live by. Many would rather suffer in silence than tell staff they are feeling sick for fear it would result in a quarantine and all programming being suspended."[21] Inmates in Saskatoon and Prince Albert, frustrated by a lack of access to physical and mental health supports and cleaning and PPE supplies to prevent transmission, staged a hunger strike (euphemistically termed "tray refusal" by the ministry) that ultimately led to changes in the protocols and treatment of the inmates during the outbreak.[22] "Before the hunger strike, our relationship to the guards was marked by continuously having things taken away from us. After our action, they started giving us more things: increased canteen, masks and cleaning supplies. All the things they were supposed to be giving us, including respect," wrote Cory, who had led the effort in Saskatoon.[23] Despite these improvements, the virus had already spread through the facility. There have been dozens of outbreaks among guards and inmates at Saskatchewan prisons since then, adding to the toll of hospitalized patients and increasing pressure on the health system, not to mention endangering the lives of those the state should be rehabilitating and protecting, not placing in harm's way.

The National Advisory Committee on Immunization and the SHA's expert panel both recommended prisons as priority settings in the second stage of the vaccine rollout. During the third wave, at a time when there were major outbreaks in Regina prisons, the Sask Party government chose to ignore this advice. When we asked about this in the legislature, the minister of justice yelled across the aisle, "Who would you take off the list?"[24] Rather than following evidence-based guidelines designed to reduce the loss of life and pressure on public health, the ministry over-rode the advice of national experts and their own officials. This rhetoric sought to pit the general public against a group of people that is seen as less deserving of medical treatment or humane conditions. It's a strategy that discards evidence in favour of division and distraction, based not on who is more vulnerable but who is seen as more politically valuable.

The lack of support for people released from corrections was further highlighted by the death of Kimberly Squirrel. Kimberly froze to death that February after being discharged from Pine Grove Correctional Centre in Prince Albert.[25] People are released from custody into home-lessness, frequently without connections to medical care, without any source of income, or – in the case of Kimberly – without even proper winter clothing. Inmates are frequently left to their own devices despite the high likelihood of reoffending or relapsing into increasingly danger-ous drug use.

While participating in a rally to support Prairie Harm Reduction, Saskatchewan's first safe consumption site, Cory described a near-miss event where he had nearly died of an overdose a year earlier. He spoke of how, if he had a safe place to go, he would feel less shame and not be using alone.[26] Jason Mercredi, former executive director of Prairie Harm Reduction, spoke to me at the time of how COVID had brought a "perfect storm of toxic drug trade, lack of access to services, lack of access to mental health supports, lack of access to basic things like food, public washrooms." More toxic and unpredictable fentanyl was on the streets and overdose deaths were on the rise. Government officials had presented documents showing that safe consumption sites would save lives and money by decreasing overdoses and transmission of HIV.[27] Nonetheless, the Sask Party, sensitive to the criticism of those who feel that harm reduction encourages drug use, has repeatedly chosen not to fund the program.[28] The site has been able to stay open due to successful fundraising campaigns, selling T-shirts, bunnyhugs, and coffee mugs to keep the lights on, but leadership is uncertain how long that generosity will last. In the meantime, the services provided appear to be making a difference; in 2021, there were half as many overdose deaths in Saskatoon as in Regina, where similar programs are not available.[29]

In June 2021, Cory died at the age of thirty-eight.[30] It wasn't COVID-19 that took Cory Cardinal's life. He was released from prison in April 2021 and was making efforts to get his life back on track, including spending time at the Calder Centre. Unable to get a safe place to stay, he turned to the street and to using again. He had made himself a shelter in the window well of a Saskatoon building, covering it with cardboard for shade and some privacy. He was found there one morning, another victim of drug poisoning. His sister, Lauren, told the CBC that, "if there had been a supervised consumption site operating 24/7 in the city, he may have had a safe place and would still be alive today."[31]

Cory may have been alone when he died, but he certainly wasn't the only person to meet such a sudden and tragic end. There was a 91 percent increase in opioid toxicity deaths in Canada in the first two years of the pandemic compared with the previous two years.[32] In Saskatchewan, we saw an increase from 179 drug toxicity deaths in 2019 (already over double the numbers from five years earlier) to 327 in 2020 and 412 in 2021. As of August 30, 2022, the province was on track to surpass that dismal record with 302 deaths and a quarter of the year left to go.[33] Over half as many people had died from overdoses as had died from COVID-19 and, while any death is a loss, overdoses are so sudden and so frequently unforeseen that they leave an added sense of emptiness in the lives of surviving families. And, just as for each person that dies from COVID there are many more who got sick or are still dealing with long-term effects, the daily struggles of people with addictions and the lack of meaningful supports to address them adds up to a tremendous burden.

Whether it's the failure to take the pending fourth wave seriously or to address the overdose and addictions crisis, the same principles are at play. An evidence-based approach to policy that uses health outcomes as a guide would dictate different choices, ones that would leave more people alive and well. Messages of intolerance toward those who have found themselves in trouble with the law or dealing with substance dependency may be more popular than investing dollars in getting them help. Declaring the pandemic over despite clear evidence to the contrary may be an easier sell than continued sacrifices. So long as the politically easy and expedient trumps what is wise and effective, so long as leaders put political gain ahead of people's lives, we will continue to spend more to get worse results.

The Dam Breaks

Jessica Bailey first learned her kidneys were failing in 2018. She needed a kidney transplant and had managed to find someone who was willing to be a donor. She was waiting to be called with a surgery date sometime in September 2021 when the organ donation program was suspended indefinitely.[1] There were too many patients in Saskatchewan hospitals with COVID, and elective and essential surgeries were being shut down. Jessica was left without hope. She was devastated when the delay resulted in her losing her donor and she was back to square one, having to start the matching process over again. The suspension of the service meant that not even this step was occurring anymore. During the time the program was suspended, there were dozens of opportunities for organ collection and donation.[2] By March 2022 her doctors had put her on palliative care and she had been removed from the transplant list because her health was too poor for her to be eligible for surgery.[3]

Graham Dickson and Laura Weins had just started to get help for their infant daughter, Helen, when it was suddenly taken away. They learned they were expecting Helen just as the provincial emergency was declared in March 2020. When she was just a few months old, they realized she wasn't meeting her milestones the way other kids of her age would. Given a presumptive diagnosis of cerebral palsy, they were running the gamut of constant tests, procedures, and appointments, and coming to grips with the lifelong challenges of supporting a child with disabilities.

For kids with developmental challenges, reaching their best potential is often dependent on early intervention; the sooner there is a clear diagnosis and targeted therapies, the better they will do in the long term.

In September 2021, they took Helen to one of her physical therapy sessions only to be told it was the last one. She'd been responding well to physio, occupational therapy, and speech language therapy, but now these services were cancelled indefinitely. The decision not to hire additional staff for testing and tracing meant that the specialized professionals she should have been seeing were being deployed as contact tracers, spending their days calling people with their COVID test results. "This was our only resource," Graham told me. "I've never felt so helpless before. To have that one thing taken away was incredibly frightening." As part of the larger slowdown of health services, Helen also had an MRI cancelled and was unable to get an essential eye surgery.

Today Helen is a happy, cute two-year-old girl who loves going to the swimming pool. She's still unable to sit on her own or to crawl but has started to speak a few words. She eventually did get the MRI, which is guiding the therapies she receives to be more specific to her condition. Her development has progressed much more quickly, and her mood is much better since her vision has improved with eye surgery. Graham and Laura believe the delay of her eye surgery until the summer of 2022 prolonged her suffering and discomfort. While they're happy to see some progress, they worry about the impact the inability to intervene in those crucial early months may have on Helen's abilities in the years ahead.

Having the mismanagement of COVID exclude their daughter from essential care was incredibly frustrating. "The economy was more important than my kid," Graham said, reflecting on what it must feel like for people who have been marginalized for generations, what it must be like to constantly receive the message that your government doesn't think helping you is worth the effort or the expense.

Helen's therapies were restored in November as those health care workers returned to their home departments. Graham believes the services were prioritized to return because he'd "made noise with the opposition." He was intimidated at first, not sure how it would be perceived to be asking for help. Yet Graham and Laura felt they had a responsibility, not just for Helen but for all the kids like her who were losing services. They understood that by sharing her story, they could write a different ending for her and for those less able to speak out.

Bringing people negatively impacted by government policies to the legislature to tell their stories is one of the most effective ways for opposition parties to get their message across. This usually starts when someone calls an MLA's office and asks for help, to advocate for them to access health care or another provincial program. If that advocacy is unsuccessful, either because the government refuses to help or because the policies in place exclude that person, there's a conversation about taking the issue public. When someone is ready to tell their story, the opposition invites them to the Legislative Building in Regina. Sometimes there's a special embargoed press conference before the sitting begins, sometimes their presence is kept as a surprise, revealed only when their issue is raised in question period. This work is one of the most challenging and rewarding parts of the job for an opposition caucus. Finding and supporting "validators," people who are willing and able to tell their story, is very difficult. It takes a lot of courage for an individual to stand up to the government, knowing that reprisal of some kind is entirely possible. It's nerve-wracking to face media scrutiny and hard to share one's personal struggles with the public.

Maybe because it's so hard, it's also extremely impactful. That fall session there were more people than ever willing to come forward and share their stories. Stephanie Brad from Domremy had major essential surgery cancelled twice due to staff redeployment.[4] Twenty-five-year-old Eden Janzen was in the dark about when she would have the parathyroid surgery and kidney transplant she needed.[5] Regina senior Dallas Oberik had been waiting two-and-a-half years for hip surgery only to have it cancelled.[6] Sarah Turnbull's two-year-old daughter, Blake, has spina bifida and lost her physical, occupational, and speech therapy because the therapists were doing contact tracing.[7] Nurses, family doctors, and clinical care assistants came to speak of how they were drowning with demand and unable to provide patients the care they deserved.

People were fed up with how the premier's decision to let the fourth wave overwhelm the system was denying them access to essential care,

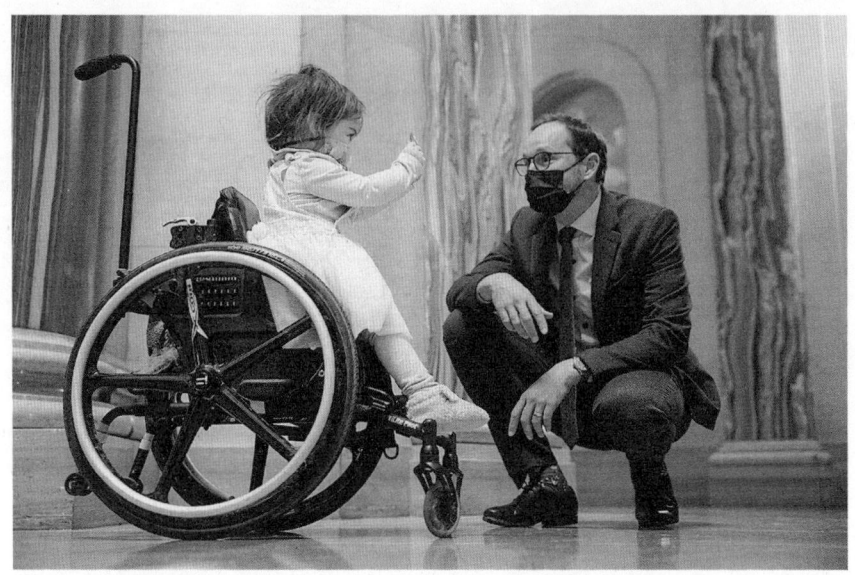

At the legislature with Blake Turnbull, who came with
her mom, Sarah, to raise awareness about cancelled therapies.
October 2021 | *Troy Fleece, republished with the express permission
of Regina Leader-Post, a division of Postmedia Network Inc.*

and they were ready to speak out. The presence of a real person willing
to tell their story makes the news, and frequently makes a difference for
that person as the government scurries to do damage control and may
get them care or even change the offending policy. The public can make
a connection to one person, one family, much more easily than they can
to statistics or policy arguments. Real people cut through the noise.

A Premier Losing Patience

September and October were two of the deadliest months of the pandemic
across Canada, with Saskatchewan suffering some of the worst outcomes
in the country. Interestingly, very few of the stories that were told publicly
at the time were of those who lost their lives. Perhaps this is because
there was a greater degree of shame or denial as many of those who died
in that period were those who had not been vaccinated. It may also be
because this was the time that the decision to pursue a mitigation strategy

Fourth Wave

– waiting until things got bad and then reacting to protect health care capacity – was proven to be a failure. Saskatchewan health care was overwhelmed. Essential procedures and services were delayed or cancelled outright, ethical triage enacted, the Armed Forces called in to help, and ICU patients loaded onto airplanes to get care halfway across the country because there wasn't room in our hospitals. The failure to protect people from COVID spilled over into a failure to protect every patient.

In that deadly fourth wave, the Prairies got hit first and worst. Outbreaks in the North started in mid-July, with over a hundred cases a day province-wide by mid-August. By mid-September, that number would rise to over 500. Despite mounting rates of transmission, the province and health authorities stayed silent. There were no COVID-related public appearances from the premier or health minister from the July 7 handshake until August 30, when the premier's message was to reject the additional measures called for by the medical health officers. Taking the pressure off left the province with our defences down. Only Alberta, where then premier Jason Kenney had taken a similar approach to the summer, experienced anything comparable.

A week after Dr. Cory Neudorf and the other medical health officers sent their letter, the leaders of the Saskatchewan Health Authority's pandemic response wrote to the premier to urge him to follow their advice. These clinical leaders, entrusted with the health care response to COVID-19, criticized the emphasis on vaccines as the only response, pointing out that "our province cannot be reliant upon a vaccine-only strategy as vaccines by themselves are not and will not be sufficient until a significantly greater proportion of our entire population is fully vaccinated."[8] They also revealed evidence that a simple measure would make a massive difference: "Provincial modelling predicts that masking may further reduce peak cases, hospitalization and ICU numbers by up to 50 per cent."[9]

This clear counsel from the province's medical leadership, with a simple change that could cut the damage of the current wave in half, had no effect. The premier said that bringing in new measures would be "unfair to the vast majority of Saskatchewan residents who have made the right decision."[10] This was a very strange idea of fairness. For one thing, the people who had done the right thing to protect themselves and those around them were more likely to want the premier to do the right thing too. Ignoring the virus and allowing the pandemic to overwhelm the health care system was the true unfairness.

Behind the scenes, Dr. Shahab was also urging the government to act. His briefing notes and recommendation to the government have not been made public, but a Global News freedom of information request in early 2023 revealed that his office had been sending stark warnings to the minister of health. A September 7 note informed the minister that "provincial vaccination coverage (two dose 69%) is insufficient to prevent acute care collapse in the absence of province-wide and targeted local measures to blunt the spread."[11] By mid-September, that collapse was underway. Case counts and hospitalizations had risen to the point that the SHA was asking the public to do their own contact tracing and announced that it was cancelling elective surgeries.[12] The province's organ donation program was suspended indefinitely a few days later.[13] Things were not going well, and the premier's attitude changed from one of dismissal to one of blame.

In a press conference on September 16, a visibly frustrated Scott Moe told the province, "We have been very patient – possibly too patient – but the time for patience is over."[14] In contrast with the conciliatory and even encouraging approach he would take with anti-vaccine movements in the coming months, he directed his criticism to those who had chosen not to get immunized, saying that "the vast majority of people in Saskatchewan have done the right thing and have grown tired of the reckless decisions of the unvaccinated that are now driving our fourth wave." A few weeks later, he said that "this pandemic is being prolonged by unvaccinated people, and there's no reason for it."[15] The blame was directed outward, as though Moe was irritated with people for listening too closely to what he'd been saying that summer. Unlike his close political ally Jason Kenney, who said, "It is now clear that we were wrong, and for that I apologize,"[16] Moe was unwilling to say sorry. He would later blame Northern communities and the prime minister for the fourth wave, citing low vaccination rates in remote communities but ignoring rates as low or lower in much of Southern Saskatchewan.[17] Not only is this pattern of punching down and pointing the finger instead of taking responsibility for the choices made far from admirable, it can also lead to reluctance for leaders to change course when a new approach is clearly needed.

On that day in mid-September, the province announced the long-overdue reintroduction of required indoor masking and a new requirement that people present proof of vaccination or a negative COVID test in the last seventy-two hours for access to restaurants and bars, entertainment venues, indoor fitness centres, and gyms. The latter would not come into effect until two weeks later. It's reasonable that new policies take time to implement. However, previous decisions to rule the idea out, as Moe had done less than a week earlier, saying that "it is not the government's role to line people up and say 'you are going to take this needle if you are going to live in this society,'"[18] not only increased resistance to this now necessary measure but also prevented any advance preparation.

Mandatory vaccination, whether for employment, education, or entry into particular venues, is an inherently controversial and delicate decision. The ethical question of insisting on a medical choice for access to normal parts of public life is not one to be taken lightly. There comes a time, however, when the greater good demands difficult choices be made. The question here is whether the necessity of mandating vaccines could have been avoided if previous steps taken had been less divisive, with a less dismissive approach prior to its implementation. What is clear is that for many Saskatchewan people, the introduction of the "higher bar" Neudorf had described was enough to motivate them to get their shots. In the first two weeks after the introduction of the proof-of-vaccination policy, the provincial rate of new vaccination was double what it had been in the preceding weeks.[19]

The problems in the Prairies attracted national attention, with Prime Minister Trudeau criticizing the approach on the federal election campaign trail and expressing sympathy for those who, despite having made the choice to get vaccinated, were still dealing with the economic and health fallout of Moe's and Kenney's choices.[20] Canadian Medical Association president Dr. Katharine Smart, originally from Saskatchewan, wrote: "We are now witnessing an unprecedented health care crisis in Alberta and Saskatchewan – and patients and health workers are experiencing unfathomable choices and consequences. Early relaxation of public health measures has left two crumbling health care systems in their wake and the dire realities are now in full view."[21] She went on to call for a "firebreaker" of aggressive public health measures in Saskatchewan and Alberta to "curb the rate of mortality, support workers, and start addressing the consequences of patients whose care is now on hold indefinitely."[22]

Saskatchewan's Wild West approach to public health had also been seen by extreme anti-health elements across Canada. Maxime Bernier, leader of the far-right People's Party of Canada (PPC), chose to host his election night celebration in Saskatchewan, citing the lack of mask rules as one of the factors. By election day there was a mask mandate in place, but his party's supporters held a large gathering in a Saskatoon hotel that flouted those public health rules and contributed to another outbreak.[23] One of the PPC candidates, prominent anti-vax activist Mark Friesen, would be admitted to hospital in Saskatoon shortly after and later flown, at great public expense, to Toronto to be treated for a disease he'd been advocating we take less seriously.[24] This pro-COVID extremism would move from the fringes to the mainstream of conservative politics in the months ahead.

September saw 90 deaths from COVID in Saskatchewan. In October, 156 people would die, in November another 76. This is the long tail of damage from decisions made in July and August. Acting late meant more pain for longer. It meant the highest death rate in Canada and it meant harder restrictions and more economic damage. It meant hospitals were still full from the fourth wave when the fifth started. The "Great Saskatchewan Summer" was over and the "fall and winter of misery" had arrived. After refusing federal help offered a month earlier, the province finally accepted military support in the middle of October, with the Canadian Armed Forces sending fifteen critical nurses and other medical personnel to spend a month helping in Regina ICUs.[25]

In the middle of that crest of death and hospitalizations, Scott Moe, pressed by veteran CBC journalist Stefani Langenegger, refused to take any responsibility or apologize, though he did say that he was "sorry that we have experienced those slowdowns here in the province."[26] He continued the pattern of downplaying his own responsibility, answering his own rhetorical question when talking to CBC Saskatoon's Leisha

Grebinski: "Should have the province [sic] moved a week, possibly 10 days earlier? You know, with the hindsight that we have now, I think we likely should have." As Langenegger pointed out, the public letter from the medical health officers – which followed on advice given privately much earlier – was released on August 26, three full weeks prior to Moe's change of course on masking and proof of vaccination.

The same day we learned of Saskatchewan patients being sent to Ontario ICUs was the day Dr. Shahab broke down while speaking with the media. By that time, the system was cracking under the pressure of COVID-19. People who had been very cautious became much clearer in their critique of the government's approach, including leaders in the SHA like Dr. Kevin Wasko or chief medical officer Dr. Susan Shaw. The presenters at that week's Physician Town Hall revealed that Saskatchewan had the highest death rate and the highest rate of patients in ICUs in the country. Modelling showed this level of "unsustainable census" in ICUs persisting for months unless gathering restrictions were brought in. Prior to his moment of emotion, Dr. Shahab was pressed on whether he was recommending gathering limits or not. He said it was "up to government" to disclose details of his recommendations. Those recommendations have never been disclosed. Side-by-side headlines on the CBC reading "Chief medical health officer says Sask. gov't needs to look at expanding reach of COVID measures"[27] and "Sask. premier says additional health measures not fair to those who have been vaccinated"[28] sent mixed messages to the public and revealed some of the internal conflict. We can read between the lines and imagine what was likely recommended, but at the end of the day it was Scott Moe's decision. He chose to say no to the measures needed to get the fourth wave under control.

Exporting Trauma

Dr. Shahab was moved to tears in the press conference. Ken Roth cried all the way to Ottawa. Ken has, in his own words, "been through hell and back." Ken is Métis, originally from Buffalo Narrows, Saskatchewan. His wife of forty-five years, Lorraine, is a member of the Clearwater River Dene Nation. They've raised four kids and a pile of grandkids in La Loche, where Ken worked for over forty years for the village. Before he got sick, he ran the water treatment plant and was proud to be making sure the people of La Loche had clean water to drink. He's a dedicated volunteer, serving on the search and rescue team for decades and as the town's volunteer fire chief for thirty-five years. In the summer of 2020, when La Loche was the site of the province's first bad outbreak, he was chair of the board of the local Friendship Centre, helping to coordinate distributing food and other support to the community when the North was locked down.

In July 2021 he missed an appointment to get his first COVID-19 vaccine when he drove to Saskatoon for a Métis Nation–Saskatchewan meeting. He and his family decided to take advantage of their having already come south and keep going for a much-needed break in Banff. He started to cough and feel sick in Drumheller, Alberta. By the time they reached Calaway Park on the outskirts of Calgary, he was barely conscious and had to be taken to Foothills Hospital, where he was admitted with COVID pneumonia. He's been told that he called family and friends to tell them he was being put under, but he doesn't remember that at all.

While he was at Foothills, his family was told to say goodbye, that he was going to die, and it was time to withdraw life support. Lorraine, who was with him every step of his brutal journey, and their daughter said no. His family held on, and so did he, eventually – with the help of insurance to cover the $20,000 transport bill – being transferred back to Saskatoon. A month later he woke up in Saint Paul's Hospital in Saskatoon, breathing through a tracheotomy tube in his neck and on dialysis because his kidneys had shut down, only to be told he was being flown to Ottawa.

Saskatchewan's ICUs were full. By September 23, there were sixty COVID patients in those ICUs. For comparison, that's the total number of hospital beds in Regina in normal times. By October 12, that number would be eighty, two more than the total number of ICU beds in the entire province. Triage of patients had already been underway to some degree for weeks, and as we entered the provincial ICU pressure "red zone" in October, it was being "widely applied."[29] I couldn't help but think that, had my dad come in with his stroke then instead of in April, it is very unlikely he would have had his surgery. A seventy-four-year-old man with a major intracranial bleed and a very low chance of recovery?

He would have never made it to the operating room that fall. Instead of seeing him visit with his grandkids months later, we'd have been doing what so many families had to do, trying to figure out how to hold a funeral by Zoom. The ICUs were so full that not only were those with a low likelihood of recovery being turned away, the patients who were in our ICUs were being sent away.

On October 20, Dr. Michael Warner, head of critical care at Michael Garron Hospital in Toronto, tweeted: "We will accept a #covid19sk ICU patient on Thurs at our hospital. Ontario has capacity because of sensible public health policies. Sask needs to implement gathering restrictions & eliminate 72h negative test in lieu of vax loophole. Policies are better than relying on planes."[30] This was initially denied by Saskatchewan provincial leadership, but ultimately it was confirmed that six patients were being transferred to Ontario.[31] There appeared to be some political interference, as shortly after, the same Ontario physician tweeted that further transfers had been cancelled.[32] This upset the already overstressed medical teams even more since, much as they didn't want to be sending patients out of province, they knew it was necessary. Upon learning about this confusion and apparent backtracking, Saskatoon intensivist Dr. Hassan Masri told the *StarPhoenix,* "We are at a point in the ICU where patient care is getting to the point that it is not safe. It is sub-standard compared to what our patients deserve."[33]

Saskatchewan physicians and the public were rightly upset to be learning about these transfers through an Ontario doctor's Twitter account rather than a straightforward message from the province. But the way Ken found out he was being transferred was worse. He described it to me as "awful." "My family was all here. They came in and said, 'you're leaving.'" He asked to talk to his family first but was told there was no time, he had to leave right then. That's when things really hit him. "When I was a little boy, six years old, they did the same thing," he said, talking about how he was taken from his mother in Buffalo Narrows to the residential school in Prince Albert. "This felt like the same trip. It hurt me so much. I cried all the way to Ottawa." We had heard so much that summer about the retraumatizing effects of the discovery of unmarked graves at residential schools across Canada, and here was a survivor reliving that pain as he was once again taken away from his family.

Ken's family drove all the way to Ottawa to see him, though most couldn't go into the hospital due to visiting restrictions. A few days later they had to turn around and drive back as, after a week in Ottawa, he was sent back to Saskatoon with no more warning on the way back than he'd had on the way out.

Back in Saskatoon, his doctor apologized to him for the way he was moved. He stayed at Saint Paul's for months, fighting his way through two bouts of hospital-acquired pneumonia. At Saskatoon City Hospital he suffered a bladder injury after a medical procedure. He was finally discharged home 378 days after he was first admitted.

The cost of keeping a patient in the hospital for over a year, with all of that transport and specialized care, is practically incalculable. The cost to Ken is obvious. He's now back in La Loche, where he's dealing with the after-effects of his illness. He's starting to be able to walk on his own, and while he no longer needs oxygen he is still short of breath. He hasn't been able to get back to work and is struggling financially. He's grateful for the support, prayers, and care he's received, but also says it's been "hard on my mind and on my soul." He's still having some very hard days and finds it challenging to tell others just what it's been like. "If you never got it like I did, you don't realize it."

While Ken's story was particularly remarkable, he was one of dozens of patients who spent months in the hospital.[34] The cost of that care, in quality of life and in real dollars, reveals the bankruptcy of arguments that the cure of preventing widespread infection with COVID through sensible public health measures was worse than the disease.

Protection Polarized

The rise in cases and lack of action prompted medical health officers (MHOs) to write Moe again on October 21. This time Dr. Neudorf and his fellow MHOs called for "stopgap measures" via a provincial health order. These included gathering restrictions; expanded proof of vaccination without the seventy-two-hour negative test option; clear government messaging on reducing contacts, working from home, and getting vaccinated; adopting the remainder of the August 26 recommendations on testing and tracing; and transparency with modelling and other data.[35]

These recommendations were supported by the Saskatchewan Medical Association and by Dr. Shahab, who said they were "all important steps that we should consider, and they're closely aligned with many recommendations that I made to government."[36]

Returning to the legislature, we asked for Dr. Shahab's recommendations to be released; the government refused. We pointed out how they had ignored the previous MHO letter and called for an emergency debate to examine the second letter and implement the recommendations. In response, the minister of education latched on to one recommendation, on expanding proof of vaccination for access to schools for school staff, students twelve and older, and households of unvaccinated students under twelve,[37] an admittedly controversial idea, but one that had also been requested by the Saskatchewan Teachers' Federation.

Instead of debating the pros and cons of this and the other public health measures presented, this was used as a "gotcha" moment. The minister of education, Dustin Duncan, ramped up the rhetoric, with us as opposition and these public health experts from the SHA being, as Murray Mandryk quipped, "misrepresented by career politicians who debased valid, professional advice with dishonest rhetoric about doctors wanting to kick kids out of school."[38] This became the talking point for the entire legislative session; whenever we raised the issues of public health measures, overwhelmed hospitals, and patients sent to Ontario, the answer was that we shouldn't listen to the province's MHOs because they wanted to kick kids out of school. It's a small example of the "big lie," the increasingly dominant form of political discourse where, no matter how ridiculous, the strategy is to repeat something terrible about your opponents loudly and confidently until it drowns out any rational argument. These cheap political games are not just abstract theatre – they have real-world effects.

Mahli and I continued to help out with vaccine clinics, including at our son's school in Saskatoon, where I had the pleasure of giving our eldest his first COVID vaccine. With his permission, I shared a photo and encouraged families to go out and get their shots. It was nice to be able to ignore the polarization for a moment and focus on something that would help us move past restrictions and isolation and toward protection for kids and the people around them.

By choosing to make children's vaccination a focus of partisan friction rather than collective action, the Sask Party contributed to greater vaccine hesitancy among parents. In the legislature Duncan refused, despite being asked repeatedly, to encourage people to get their children vaccinated. He would later step in and prevent local schools from requiring vaccination for participation in extracurricular activities, even when those schools were in outbreak and that measure was put in place with the recommendation of the local medical health officer.[39] The message was clear: children's immunization had become controversial and whatever the public health impact, the Sask Party saw their safer political bet as being with those worried more about the vaccine than the virus.

Health Minister Paul Merriman took things further, changing a long-standing practice of parental consent for in-school vaccinations and instead requiring that parents be present at any school clinics for COVID-19 vaccinations.[40] It's hard to describe just how extraordinary this move was. This year my son got the HPV and meningococcal vaccine at school along with his Grade 6 classmates, just as thousands do every year. There is no reason that the COVID vaccines should be treated any differently. If parents didn't want the vaccine given at school, they could simply choose not to sign the form. It's that easy. What isn't easy is getting off work to be present at the school to accompany your kid for their vaccines. Earlier in the pandemic the government had allotted sick time coverage for individuals wanting to get their shots. Despite our requests for this policy to be extended to give coverage to parents and caregivers accompanying others to get their shots, the government chose to eliminate the program instead.

Compare this to Newfoundland and Labrador, where, rather than being used as a wedge issue, children's vaccination was universally promoted with a robust public health communication strategy. Chief medical health officer Dr. Janice Fitzgerald, who had gained public trust with clear, consistent messaging, held press conferences on child vaccination options and sent letters to parents promoting opportunities for immunization. An advertising campaign promoted the ways in which vaccination would help children to safely reunite with their grandparents.

The province wanted to ride the wave of excitement at vaccine approval and have as many children as possible vaccinated before Christmas.

They were able to move quickly due to a strong public health nursing system developed as the island fought tuberculosis and polio through the last century. Bookings for all five-to-eleven-year-olds were open as soon as the vaccine was approved, mass clinics were operating within days, and school-based clinics opened across Newfoundland and Labrador. As of October 2022, 89 percent of children aged five to eleven in Newfoundland had received their first dose, compared with only 51 percent in Saskatchewan.[41] Newfoundland and Labrador chose to put children's health first and use their strengths to get kids their shots. The Sask Party chose to make children's vaccination a wedge issue to deflect attention away from the disastrous management of the fourth wave. It's a tremendous example of the difference between governing for people and governing for power.

Health Care in Crisis

Politicizing children's vaccines is a striking example of cynical politics at play, but of course we are never free from politics, between or within parties. When I think of that fourth wave, it feels further away than some of the others. I expect that's partly a function of the incredible speed of change at the time, partly how used to COVID we'd become, and partly distraction from my own growing burnout. It's also fair to say my focus was divided between the pandemic response and issues within the NDP. A small group had chosen to push for me to be removed as leader at the provincial convention in early October. In every political party, a leader manages the tension between the idealists and the win-at-all-costs factions of their party, along with the tension between what the public already wants and what the party believes they should want. Navigating this is always a study in compromise.

Due to the rising case count, our annual party convention was all online that year. In my speech, delivered to a camera instead of a crowd of activists, I tried to fire up the members with criticism of our opponents and talk of our big plans. I also talked about how no one's mental health had been spared, mine included, and how we were all trying our best to balance challenging lives in a time of uncertainty and fear. When I think of the conflicts of this period, I try to remember the stress people were under. I recall sitting with some of my closest friends in the party that afternoon, hoping we would have the support of the members to keep fighting. As tired as I might be, it was no time to leave; I needed to at least see out the worst of the pandemic. Seventy-two percent of the delegates voted that day in favour of my continued leadership. That was high enough to stay, but low enough to leave doubt and ongoing drama.

At the same time, internal drama was playing out in the Saskatchewan Health Authority. Scott Livingstone had been serving as the chief executive officer of the SHA since it was formed from the amalgamation of twelve health regions in 2017. The SHA was meant to operate at arm's-length from the Ministry of Health, with a board appointed by the government and an Executive Leadership Team chosen by the CEO. While Dr. Shahab was the face of the government's pandemic response, his responsibility was public health orders and advice. The health system response – hospitals and clinics, drug supplies, vaccine rollout, etc. – was the work of the SHA. Throughout the first three waves of the pandemic, the ministry and the SHA seemed to speak with one voice. That started to change in the fourth wave, with the SHA sounding the alarm on social media, in press conferences, and in Physician Town Halls in ways that were jarringly different from the premier's and the health minister's downplaying of the seriousness of the situation.

The first sign that something was going seriously wrong in this relationship came on October 9. As Adam Hunter wrote for the CBC, Premier Moe's message to Saskatchewan people ahead of the Thanksgiving long weekend was not about taking extra precautions to bring down nation-leading COVID-19 cases and record hospitalizations – it was to explain a new structure aimed at coordinating pandemic response.[42] A few days earlier, Scott Livingstone had said that help from outside the province may be needed and that we were close to needing to employ medical triage procedures.[43] Now the management of the pandemic was being handed over to a newly developed Provincial Emergency Operations Centre, a combined body of the Saskatchewan Public Safety Agency, the SHA, and the Ministry of Health. This was more about controlling the message than it was about controlling the virus.

The effort to assert control over the SHA appears to have escalated from there. Scott Livingstone left the position of CEO suddenly at the

Fourth Wave

beginning of December.[44] He had been a visible representative of the pandemic response and was well respected by the public and by health care workers in the SHA. A few days later we would learn that Raynelle Wilson, a former Sask Party candidate and political operative, had been placed in a newly created vice-president role on the SHA Executive Leadership Team. Credible sources reported that Wilson's appointment, and the government interference it represented, was the last straw that led Livingstone to walk away.[45] This may seem like inside baseball but the departure of the head of the health care system in the middle of the worst wave of the pandemic because of political interference is a big deal. It says a lot about who the government was and wasn't listening to at the time, and the lengths they would go to in order to exercise control.

Losing the lead of your health system is also not a great way to kick off a massive catch-up effort in health care. The displaced surgeries, primary care, screening, and specialist visits during the periods that clinics and hospitals were either proactively shuttered or overwhelmed by COVID will mean increased demand on clinical services for years to come. As of April 2022, over 35,000 people – nearly 3 percent of the population – were waiting for surgery in Saskatchewan, up by over a third from before the pandemic.[46] No family doctors in Saskatoon are accepting new patients.[47] The story is the same across the country, where talk of a national health care crisis gets louder every day. In June, Canadian Medical Association president Katharine Smart spoke at the time of a system "collapsing around us."[48] Frustratingly, the fall 2022 meeting between federal health minister Jean-Yves Duclos and his provincial counterparts ended early over a dispute on whether new federal dollars should come with expectations.[49] The eventual health funding deal in February 2023 saw $46.2 billion flowing to the provinces over ten years.[50] However, with no real strings attached and only 58 percent of that money required to be spent on health care, there is a high risk of repeating the pattern of earlier health accords that did not buy real change.

Our health system has been redlined for years, with increasingly louder cries for reform. A great deal will be said and written about the exact actions that need to be taken around physician credentials, team-based care, staffing levels, and training opportunities. These are important conversations to have and deserve our attention. They are secondary, however, to the foundational principle of the continued existence and improvement of a single-payer, publicly funded health care system that serves people based on their medical need. One of the things I love most about being a physician in Canada is that when I see a patient in front of me, I get to ask them how they're feeling, not how they're paying.

While the distribution of service is by no means universal or equitable, that underlying principle of care based on need, not ability to pay, makes a massive difference in the quality, accessibility, and affordability of medical care for all Canadians. The current crisis, however, is the kind that governments of a certain stripe will be keen not to waste. We see this already underway in Saskatchewan, with the government announcing private surgical centres as the solution to surgical backlogs,[51] and an Alberta premier with long-standing plans to incorporate more direct patient payment for basic health services.[52] While there have always been private providers in Medicare, we should be very wary of "new models" that charge patients directly, violating the Canada Health Act. This moment demands reform and major investment, and we must make sure that those funds and those plans are used to bring our public health care system back from the brink, not push it over.

Fifth Wave

DECEMBER 2021 – APRIL 2022

> All I can say is that on this earth
> there are pestilences and there are victims –
> and as far as possible one must refuse to be
> on the side of the pestilence.

– Albert Camus, *The Plague*

Total cases in Canada	1.97 million
Total cases in Saskatchewan	Unknown due to changes in testing and reporting
Deaths from COVID in Canada	8,889
Deaths from COVID in Saskatchewan	397

Provincial Public Health Measures

December 30, 2021	PCR confirmation of rapid antigen test no longer recommended Isolation requirements reduced to five days for vaccinated
February 7, 2022	PCR testing no longer available to general public
February 13, 2022	Proof of vaccination policy ends
February 28, 2022	All public health measures lifted, including masking

Putting It Mildly

Two years after the state of emergency was called in March 2020, a hush fell over the Saskatchewan Legislative Building. All the staff and MLAs had gone home and the building was again off limits to the public. But this time it wasn't the virus shutting things down, it was the people who didn't believe we should fight it.

Concrete blocks and security barred the entrance to the Saskatchewan legislature in February as Sergeant-at-Arms Terry Quinn and his team prepared for protests. In a moment of surprising candour, a Saskatchewan Party backbencher I met in the lobby said to me, "I don't know what they're protesting, Scott's giving them everything they want," referring to the premier's love letter a few days earlier to the so-called freedom convoy, where he pointed to their efforts as the reason "why, in the not-too-distant future, our government will be ending our proof of negative test/proof of vaccination policy in Saskatchewan."[1]

Despite the premier's prophylactic capitulation, admirers of the protests that had paralyzed downtown Ottawa were planning similar actions across the country, including in Regina. Fortunately, Mr. Quinn and his legislative security team and Regina Police Chief Evan Bray were way ahead of them, setting up blockades to protect the legislature. The protesters who were rebuffed had every reason to be surprised by this; after all, the premier had been encouraging them to make their voices heard. Terry and his team's ability to protect the people's house and prevent the kind of protracted anti-government, anti–public health occupation that had gridlocked the nation's capital for days appears to have had political ramifications. In the next session, the Sask Party chose to pass legislation handing the role of protecting the assembly over from the independent sergeant-at-arms to a private security force that answered to a cabinet minister.

Falling for Falsehoods

A year earlier, in May 2021, Premier Scott Moe had some welcome strong words on vaccines, saying to those who hadn't yet gone for their shot, "We're not asking you to storm the beaches of Normandy. All we're asking you to do is to go in and to get a tiny needle in your arm."[2] That fall, he blamed the unvaccinated for the fourth wave, saying he was losing patience with their "reckless decisions."[3] Shortly after, he sent a clear message to the anti-vax movement, saying: "The evidence is clear. Vaccines do work. We listened to the doctors. We listened to the experts. Stop listening to all the nonsense that is out there on social media," and "Believing in and spreading anti-vaccine conspiracy theories is actually contributing to people dying from COVID."[4] This straight talk was a welcome response to a growing problem.

By December, his tone shifted as he called on people to stop "stigmatizing the unvaccinated." Given that he had been doing just that with some of his earlier statements, this could have been a positive intervention and course correction. Attacking people for their choices is not likely to change their behaviour. It can, however, lead people to use judgmental language or even consider the unethical idea of denying care for those not immunized.[5] Moe was right to stop the stigmatizing language and encourage others to do the same.

In the weeks ahead, however, the premier's language took a strange turn. Despite modelling showing an exponential rise in new cases, he dismissed the idea of gathering restrictions in response to December's growing Omicron wave, not wanting to "take away your personal freedoms." In February 2022, he described the proof-of-vaccination policies of the Delta wave as having "effectively created two classes of citizens. To my knowledge, this province has never done anything like that before in our history, for any vaccine or for any other reason for that matter."[6]

This would be echoed a few months later by newly elected Alberta premier Danielle Smith, who said those who hadn't been vaccinated against COVID were "the most discriminated-against group that I've ever witnessed in my lifetime."[7] These ahistorical statements were rightly pilloried, displaying as they did shocking ignorance of glaring examples of classifications and discrimination such as Indian residential schools, the reserve pass system, or even the R that was still on Saskatchewan health cards of Registered Indians at the time of Moe's comments.

So what happened? Why did the premier's attitude to anti-vaxers go from excessively judgmental to sycophantic in a matter of months? We'll likely never know what opinion polling, pressure from his own MLAs, or fear of the rise of a vote-splitting right-wing alternative may have contributed to this shift, but one event stood out. Nadine Ness is the founder of Unified Grassroots, an organization that had joined People's Party of Canada (PPC) candidate Mark Friesen in an unsuccessful effort to obtain a court injunction against vaccine mandates in September. In November, the group held a candlelight vigil after Health Canada's approval of the Pfizer-BioNTech vaccine for children aged five to eleven, to "pray for and support the children and families" that would supposedly be harmed by the vaccine.[8] Ness had started to gain a following for her YouTube videos that criticized the province's COVID measures. After posting a video titled "A Message to Scott Moe" that garnered a thousand views, her next video showed that Scott got the message. Ness revealed that the premier spent an hour on the phone listening to her complaints and theories.

Contrast this with the many people Moe had refused to meet or acknowledge, such as Tristen Durocher during his time in Wascana Park, any of the hundreds of doctors who wrote to him multiple times, or patients like Jessica Bailey and Helen Dickson who had come to the legislature. For them he had no time, but for someone who spread conspiracy theories and false information about vaccines, he was keen not only to pick up the phone but also to change his tune.

Ness took to Facebook to take credit for the shift to the language of "not stigmatizing," which came in the days following the call. Two days after Sask Party MLAs attended a Unified Grassroots Zoom presentation, the premier announced that Saskatchewan would be the only Canadian province not to introduce gathering limits during the Omicron wave. Ness boasted that this was connected to her advocacy,[9] and a Unified Grassroots phone blitz to MLA offices in January may have contributed to the premier's commitment to remove all measures at the end of that month. The premier went from "We listened to the doctors. We listened to the experts"[10] to listening to a fringe group promoting the very misinformation he said in October was killing people.

This is cause for reflection for those who have been trying to advocate for evidence-based responses to COVID, or a provincial opposition that has sought to amplify those voices. A report from the Canadian Council of Academies estimates that vaccine hesitancy caused by misinformation cost 2,800 Canadian lives and over $300 million in hospital expenses between March and November of 2021.[11] Yet despite the obvious damage caused, many politicians continue to cater to the groups peddling these lies. How do you break through with messages based on facts when ignorance or outright falsehoods are winning the day? The growing tide of misinformation presents a substantial challenge for those who want to see governments enact evidence-based policies with the best interests of Canadians in mind.

Omicron Changes the Game

A new variant of SARS-CoV-2 first detected in late November 2021 in South Africa and Botswana was named Omicron, after the fifteenth letter of the Greek alphabet. Omicron appeared to be a descendant of earlier versions of the virus rather than a mutation of the Alpha or Delta variants. The emergence of new variants in parts of the world that had been less able to afford or effectively distribute the most effective vaccinations further underlined how, when the disease is global, the response must be global. Not only was the failure of wealthy countries to prioritize access to vaccines for low- and middle-income countries a factor in the health disasters in many poorer nations, it also made the pandemic worse in the places with the resources to fight it.

Coming on the heels of a fourth wave that was only starting to fade, Omicron spread much more quickly than previous versions of the virus and evaded the protection of the available vaccines much more effectively.

Hospitals across Canada were still full and many of those patients would be there for weeks or months to come. Saskatchewan was at particular risk, still dealing with the highest rates of ICU admission in the country. We simply couldn't afford another crush of COVID patients. Our first call as the opposition was to expand access to booster doses as early assessments showed an increase in protection from infection and severe outcomes with a third dose.[12] The first case of Omicron would arrive in the province a few days later. By the middle of December, the province agreed to expand boosters but took no other actions to prevent the spread of Omicron.

Just before Christmas, Scott Moe posted a video in which he talked about Omicron cases being "mild." This was incautious to say the least. The early data offered some hope that the risk to an individual of a serious outcome from Omicron was less than from Delta, but it was far too early to be giving people a false sense of confidence. Only two days earlier, the province had released modelling showing cases, hospitalizations, and ICU admissions rising steeply in the weeks ahead. Worse than this premature declaration of mildness was the absence of an important disclaimer. If a smaller percentage of the people who catch a disease get sick, but way more people catch the virus, the result is still many people winding up in hospital or dying. This "milder" version of the virus would go on to kill 143 Saskatchewan people in February and another 136 in March, the deadliest two-month period since the beginning of the pandemic.

Omicron truly did change the game. The vaccine escape and increased transmissibility led to daily case numbers so high that the existing approach, both to reporting and to fighting the virus, was obsolete. The COVID-zero or suppression policies that were the most effective with earlier variants were now no longer viable. Whether or not PCR testing and reporting of daily cases were feasible or desirable, the numbers meant little in comparison to previous waves. And people were exhausted. Pandemic fatigue had set in long before, but the brutal experience of the fourth wave had finished off what little patience people had left. Provincial messaging didn't help, with Scott Moe telling people, "Remember when this first started, so very long ago? Government measures were supposed to last, I think, two weeks. Well, it's been two years," which fed into the fatigue and sense of being wronged rather than providing leadership to guide people to a place of sustained effort.[13]

It may not make sense to lose patience with a microbe, to be fed up with doing what's necessary for people's health, but that's where people were and the people who should have been leading were following instead. It's all very well to be "done with COVID," but the virus decides when it's done with us. We can try to take the least disruptive and most effective steps to protect those who continue to be vulnerable to the immediate and long-term effects of the pandemic, or we can accept avoidable death and disability. Those are the choices, whatever our feelings may be.

But feelings matter. Human beings make decisions based on emotions and beliefs, not cold logic. Sometimes we respond to feelings that provoke action: fear, sympathy, anger, infatuation. We also experience emotions that move us to stop acting. In the case of COVID-19, worry over our own health and solidarity with those at risk of getting sick moved us to spend public dollars and alter our lives. As time wore on, like fight-or-flight sympathetic responses, that level of commitment to change couldn't be maintained, at least not without a different story being told. The disappointment of discovering that, because of the Omicron variant, vaccines were no longer the final answer we'd hoped for made that even harder.

The first twenty-four deaths over the first six months of the pandemic were a cause of great public discussion and grief. In the winter of 2022, twenty-two people were dying a week and we called it over. Human beings are designed to adapt to even the most strenuous circumstances. Historian Dan Gardner describes how "repeated exposure to a stimulus gradually reduces its salience."[14] People adjusted to the 1918 influenza even though it continued to kill in high numbers for years. They adjusted to the noise of industrial workplaces or to the carnage of vehicular accidents. This inurement to threats is natural; we can't constantly be in a state of alarm – that level of vigilance is too exhausting and would deaden our ability to respond to new stimuli. Over time we go through a process of habituation – simply accepting something destructive as a part of life – and adaptation, changing the way we operate to decrease the effect without disrupting life to an incapacitating degree. Traffic laws, regulations for automobile manufacturers, and workplace safety standards were resisted when introduced but soon became part of the landscape. When it comes to COVID, the same process is underway: what adaptations – e.g., mask use during high seasons, regular vaccinations, etc. – we will keep versus what measures are simply too disruptive to maintain. That's why it is so important to be targeted, evidence-based, and nuanced in both measures and messages, and why the failure to do so created space for those who would advocate against keeping people safe.

Into this mix of pandemic fatigue arose another phenomenon, what Charleston University medical history professor Jacob Steere-Williams calls "endemic fatalism."[15] This is the idea that COVID is here to stay, and everyone will get it, so there's no point trying to prevent transmission or even monitor the disease. Steere-Williams tracked the public uses of the word "endemic" and saw an enormous change in the frequency and type of use in early 2021. "Endemic" can mean locally contained or widespread and recurrent. The latter, as applied to seasonal influenza, is one of the potential futures for COVID: a disease that returns annually or semi-annually with variations in its presentation and the required response. The problem is not with the term, but with the use of it to mean we can stop taking the situation seriously. To quote *Globe and Mail* health columnist André Picard, "Yes, COVID-19 is becoming endemic. But we can't buy into the delusion that is a synonym for harmless."[16]

The flu causes varying degrees of illness each year and is rightly the subject of annual public vaccination campaigns. In Mozambique, I worked alongside communities who were distributing bed nets and eliminating stagnant water because the mosquito-borne endemic illness malaria was killing their children at alarming rates. Tuberculosis is endemic to much of the world and is the single deadliest infectious disease on the planet. Endemicity is a legitimate epidemiological concept, but too many of those using the term during the fifth wave appeared to be attracted to the first three letters of the word, as though COVID's establishment as endemic was not a sign of worrisome persistence, but rather the end.

In the vacuum of uncertainty and inurement, two trends emerged: bad information and no information. Sadly, Saskatchewan found itself at the forefront of both. "Canadian premier tests positive day after rejecting COVID measures," read the headline of the *Guardian* on January 14, 2022, as our province's pandemic response was once again an international embarrassment. Two days earlier, despite climbing hospitalizations and every other province increasing their public health measures, Scott Moe had declined to enhance Saskatchewan's. In another display of contradictory messages, while chief medical health officer Dr. Saqib Shahab encouraged people to increase mask use and limit discretionary contact, Moe questioned the effectiveness of social distancing and gathering restrictions in the context of Omicron. Asked whether people should trust him or the public health officials, rather than acknowledge the disconnect he said that "they should trust themselves."[17]

Saskatchewan Union of Nurses president Tracy Zambory described the dismay of exhausted health care workers in the face of this abdication of leadership and said, with regard to the premier, "He's gambling with the system, he's gambling with people's lives, he's gambling with the fact we have a health human resource crisis on our hands that they should be well aware of."[18] The next day, Moe announced on Twitter that he had tested positive for COVID-19, notably having appeared without a mask at a number of community events and in the previous day's COVID briefing with a masked Dr. Shahab.

The incongruity between the messages of Moe and Shahab went beyond their choice of face coverings. As hospitalizations climbed, doctors were being warned through the month of January to ready themselves for major service disruptions in what might be the toughest wave yet.[19] On January 26 Dr. Shahab announced the need to "stay the course for another four to six weeks to prevent a rebound." On the same day Scott Moe went on right-wing radio to announce his plans to remove restrictions in the "next number of days." There had been not-so-subtle differences in the messages from public health leadership and political leadership throughout the pandemic, but nothing so overt. Clearly, the people in charge of the health system wanted to keep working to protect people from COVID. The people elected to represent the best interests of Saskatchewan people had entirely moved on.

In those "next number of days," the province removed the requirement for people who tested positive for COVID to self-isolate and for parents to inform schools when their kids tested positive. *Regina Leader-Post* columnist Murray Mandryk wrote in response: "The numbers on the Saskatchewan COVID-19 Dashboard are screaming right now that Premier Scott Moe and his Saskatchewan Party government should actually be doing the opposite of what they are."[20] The answer from Moe and the Sask Party? If the numbers are screaming, kill the numbers.

On February 3, 2022, Saskatchewan passed a thousand deaths from COVID-19. The government marked the occasion by announcing it would be the first province to switch from daily to weekly pandemic reporting. From February 6 on, weekly summary reports were released on Thursday afternoons, making them less able to be reported on or used as fodder for questions in the legislature. Those reports would become even more irrelevant that summer when the province switched to monthly summaries. There is a legitimate question as to the relevance of daily case counts with Omicron's massive spread, but the rates of hospitalization and death remained extremely relevant and extremely high. Instead, we were left with analysis of how much virus was found in the wastewater of the province's major cities as the only reliable source of current information.

The message from the government at the time was that we needed to learn to live with COVID. Fair enough. But learning to live with something and pretending it doesn't exist are very different. We were simultaneously told to make our own personal risk assessments while having the information required to make those assessments taken away, asked to "trust our own choices" with nothing to guide those choices. I joked at the time that, in a frozen Saskatchewan February, I was eager for spring and that if I could snap my fingers and make it spring the next day, I probably would. But if I told people winter was already over while it was still twenty-five below, if I told them we were going to read the temperature only once a week or once a month, if I told them to ditch their parkas and head outside in a T-shirt and trade their winter boots for sandals, that would be completely dishonest and irresponsible. But when it came to COVID, that's exactly what happened. The frightening thing is, it worked.

It didn't work to stop the virus. Hospitalizations were near the Delta peak at the time of the decision to stop sharing daily information. They would go on to eclipse that peak in February and reach even higher levels in April.[21] Hundreds more would die that spring with hardly a mention. It didn't work to stop the virus, but it did work to change the channel. Without reliable daily accounting of the situation, people quickly looked away. Deaths kept coming, but for most people the pandemic had passed, not because the virus was gone but because we stopped talking about it. We would hear stories that spring of people presenting to emergency dumbfounded, in disbelief that their illness could be COVID because they'd heard it was over. The decision to stop access to testing and daily reporting was panned by the opposition and by critical responses on social media and in the press, but the demand soon faded and the Sask Party proclaimed the end of information a resounding success.[22]

This is the frightening thing to me, that the lesson that Canada's far right – which is increasingly how one would have to define the Prairie conservative parties – has learned is not to do what must be done to achieve the best outcomes, but to turn off the lights as soon as possible. The political calculus won out over the moral. Whatever the issue – COVID, suicide rates, poverty, crime, employment – if the lesson is to hide and obscure the data earlier and more effectively, then the very idea of a Canada led by its people is at risk. Free and timely access to information is an essential ingredient for democracy. Shannon Gormley, writing for *Maclean's* on the prevalence of poor pandemic outcomes in dictatorships, described how "dictatorships must obscure their failure to uphold their end of the dishonest bargain they made – their failure, that is, to keep the nation secure. These regimes fear that should people discover the full extent of their failure, it is their own security that would be under threat. This may be one reason that all types of dictatorship have a negative impact on health outcomes."[23] Despite overwrought claims from either end of the political spectrum, Canada is by no means a dictatorship. That is something to be proud of, but also something to defend. That defence includes, among other factors, a truly free and independent press, fair and objective electoral laws, and an engaged and informed public. Erosion in each of those elements in recent years in Canada has accelerated since the beginning of COVID-19, and with anti-democratic currents on the rise worldwide, we should take that erosion very seriously.

Misinformation was on the rise, as were efforts to discredit legitimate research. University of Toronto professor Tara Moriarty was the lead author of a Royal Society of Canada study that examined the rates of excess deaths across the country.[24] By examining the total number of deaths in 2020 compared with the expected number from a non-pandemic year, the study showed that COVID deaths across the country were likely significantly higher than the official counts. The report suggested that as many as 6,000 COVID deaths had gone unreported across Canada between February and November 2020. In Saskatchewan, for example, nearly 700 more people died in 2020 than in 2019, the highest number of deaths in seventy-five years. However, only 153 COVID deaths were recorded. Data from Statistics Canada suggest Saskatchewan experienced 1,288 excess deaths in 2021, despite only confirming 839 COVID-related deaths.[25] Moriarty's study suggested that lack of posthumous testing (which Manitoba and Quebec, the provinces with the highest official counts of COVID deaths, perform) and deaths at home among seniors and racialized frontline workers would account for the majority of those unrecorded COVID deaths.

In response to Moriarty's report, the premier lashed out, calling it "nothing short of some of the most egregious misinformation that I've seen throughout this pandemic."[26] This would be a bizarre response to a peer-reviewed academic study, until one realizes how central downplaying the pandemic and spinning Saskatchewan's response as effective has been to the Sask Party's public narrative. When I asked about the excess deaths in the legislature, the minister of health not only showed no curiosity about what might be causing the deaths of hundreds of Saskatchewan residents if it wasn't COVID-19, he accused me of maligning the ability of doctors to fill out death certificates. It is quite revealing that, in a time of rampant, deliberate misinformation about the virus and the vaccines and other measures that can help protect us from it, what got Scott Moe hopping mad was a credible study from one of the country's most respected scientific bodies.

Not satisfied with calling out facts as misinformation, Scott Moe decided to take a turn at spreading some fake news of his own. In his strange, all-caps-riddled missive to the province's truckers, a vanishingly small percentage of whom were skipping work to go honk their horns in Ottawa, Moe wrote that "vaccination is not reducing transmission," and that "an unvaccinated trucker does not pose any greater risk of transmission than a vaccinated trucker."[27] He would later go on to make misleading statements about provincial data indicating that people who were vaccinated were actually more likely to be infected.[28]

None of these statements was true at the time and they are not true today. While the Omicron variant had a much higher rate of vaccine escape than previous versions of the virus, vaccines not only reduced the likelihood of hospitalization or death, they also still substantially reduced the likelihood of catching COVID for those who had received a booster shot. As for unvaccinated people posing no risk to others, a study from the University of Toronto showed that a greater degree of mixing between vaccinated and unvaccinated people increased the risk of infection to those who had received the vaccine.[29] Vaccination remained as important a measure as a year earlier, when the premier was touting it as "the best thing we can all do to protect ourselves and those around us and get life back to normal."[30]

So why was the premier of the province with the second-lowest rate of vaccination in the country, as the *Saskatoon StarPhoenix* headline read, "repeating falsehoods on vaccines?"[31] Murray Mandryk summed it up nicely: "The only reasonable conclusion that can be drawn is politics. Moe and other conservatives in the country obviously feel they can't contradict that loud, angry message emerging from the 'freedom' convoy – especially when it's mostly directed at Prime Minister Justin Trudeau and the federal Liberal government."[32] The convoy protesters may have occupied Ottawa for three weeks, but they have completely captured Canada's conservatives, just as the January 6 insurrectionists stormed any semblance of the pre-Trump Republican Party in the United States. The elections of Pierre Poilievre and Danielle Smith as leaders of the federal and Alberta branches of Canadian conservatives represent a dramatic shift toward a populism with a taste for conspiracy theories and authoritarianism. As for Saskatchewan, Scott Moe's Sask Party has shifted from a Liberal-Conservative coalition to a party increasingly beholden to its far-right Buffalo wing.

This was on full display with Moe's response to the convoy. Aside from the vaccine nonsense, one could be generous and say that he hadn't done his homework and didn't know what the convoy would turn into at the time he wrote his letter. That excuse was long gone with desecration of national monuments, harassment of Ottawa residents, a bizarre plan to replace the elected federal government with a committee of the speaker of the Senate, the governor general, and the people of Canada as represented by "Canada Unity," and blockades of international borders in Alberta, Manitoba, and Ontario.[33] Nonetheless, on February 9, Moe moved from supporting the protesters' objection to cross-border vaccine mandates to praising their overall mission of getting rid of public health measures; he applauded them for "getting their voices heard" and said he would "stay out of telling them what to do."[34]

Working-class people were being sold a false, flag-waving freedom by a government that has made them less free. A government that deliberately keeps wages low, rejects bills to make working conditions safer, sees government bids go to its donors, all while it becomes harder for citizens to see a doctor or ensure their kids receive a decent education, is stealing freedom, not granting it. The cynical willingness to hide behind grievances they helped create instead of leading people to the wisest response to a once-in-a-lifetime challenge is a damning indictment.

A few days after the convoy reached Ottawa, Moe went all in, prematurely ending the proof-of-vaccination policy and announcing that all public health orders would expire permanently at the end of the month. He said it was "time to heal the divisions."[35] While the echoes of the Unified Grassroots message were audible in this message, there have indeed been divisions. Around the world, debates over COVID have divided neighbours and family members. People have cut off contact with each other due to differences in beliefs and approaches to the pandemic.

This is a challenging reality to lead through and requires clear communication and courage to tell the truth. To instead cite divisions and stop sharing information about COVID, stop taking evidence-based action to protect those at risk, and minimize a danger while it is still very much present, is a failure to meet that challenge. Making choices that make more people sick is no way to heal divisions.

Bringing Work Home

More people died from COVID per day in February 2022 than in any other month of the pandemic to date. At the end of February, all public health orders in Saskatchewan came to an end. Weekly reports made it impossible to track what was really happening. Thrust into a world of rumours and guesses, with growing public pressure to just move on, we were truly on our own. Mahli and I remained extra-cautious. She was in hospital and clinic all the time and I was still doing weekly clinics at the Lighthouse. I continued to mask at the legislature, as I couldn't risk bringing anything to or from my patients, the public, or my family. Abe wore a mask to Grade 5 and Gus to pre-K.

Despite our best efforts to avoid it for ourselves and others, COVID found its way to our house as well. On the Thursday before Easter, Gus got sent home with a fever. He tested positive with a rapid antigen test that evening. He was miserable with a forty-degree temperature overnight but wasn't coughing. The next day he was sleepy and febrile. I stayed home with him and he fell asleep with his head on my chest, something he hadn't done in forever. There was no way we could isolate from a four-year-old, of course, so it was only a matter of time before the virus spread through the house.

Mahli started to feel bad that Friday. She was coughing and febrile and had a positive rapid test. She got the worst of it, in bed for days and exhausted by the slightest effort. Getting up to have a shower was like a full day's work. Abe and I were still fine, maybe a bit of sore throat, but still testing negative. Instead of going to Easter Mass, I took the boys on a mini-pilgrimage out to the Mount Carmel shrine near Humboldt, which we'd visited when doing our lockdown walkabouts in March 2020. Gus was feeling a bit better, running around with our two dogs, but then fell asleep in the car on the way home, and we were all in bed way earlier than usual.

On Monday morning, I woke up to the sound of Gus crying. I went into his room and he said he couldn't walk. He tried to get out of bed but had too much pain in his legs. His calves were sore to the touch and he couldn't even bear weight long enough to pee. Otherwise, he was his

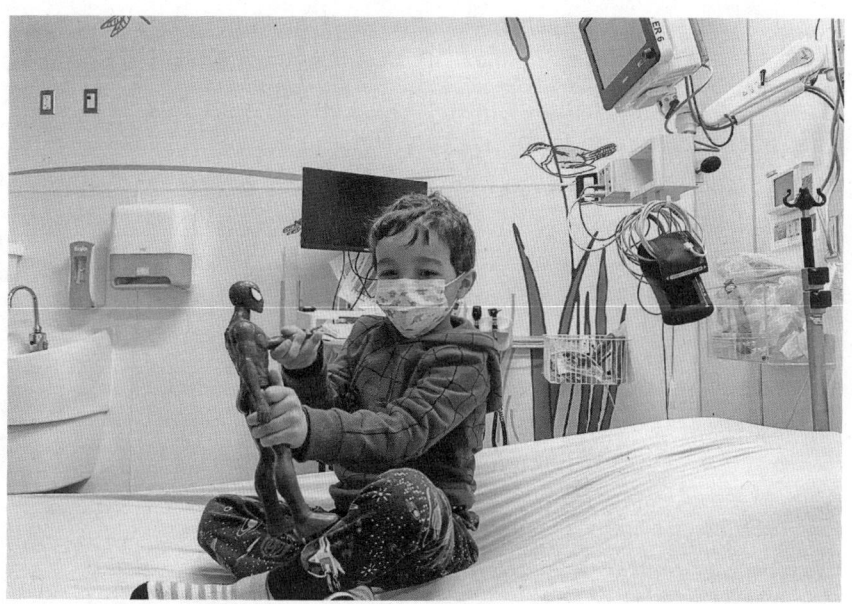

Gus in pediatric emergency with COVID-19. April 2022

good old Gussy self, full of energy, scooting around the floor and up and down the stairs. He just couldn't stand up. Luckily the holiday Monday was still quiet in the emergency room at the Children's Hospital. The pediatrician examined him and ordered some labs. Creatinine kinase (CK) levels are a sign of muscle breakdown. His CK was very high at 1400, which gave us the diagnosis of viral myositis. This means that COVID was attacking the muscles in his legs, which is painful but not dangerous in itself. The big risk is that the CK levels get so high that they damage the kidneys.

I thought back to all the messages we'd heard about kids – "schools are safe; kids don't spread COVID; if they do catch it, they don't get sick" – but I didn't have the energy to be mad about it. I just held my kid. We cuddled up to read books and watch Zootopia on my laptop while he got ibuprofen and half a litre of IV fluids. After that, he could walk with a limp and we went home with a cardboard-and-gauze contraption to keep the IV line in place so he could have another bolus of fluids the next day.

The next morning Gus was back to his usual self and got the okay from pediatric emergency to ditch the IV and skip any further bloodwork. Abe was sore and tired with a headache and was starting to lose his sense of taste; he tested positive. I was croaky and my rapid test was positive too, completing the family set. Thankfully, we were on a break from the legislature that week and I could isolate and stay home with the boys. Gus had given us a good scare, but all in all, we had it pretty easy. Mahli and I were both well protected with three shots and the boys recovered well. Since then I've noticed that we all get worse colds and I can't help but wonder if there are some lingering effects, but if we were going to get it, I'm glad it was then and not sooner.

It was a rough week, but we were lucky and I'm grateful for that. And it's tempting, as I think so many of us have done, to extrapolate what turned out to be a minor illness for yourself to something not being a big problem in general. In the week we were sick, there were 417 people in Saskatchewan hospitals with COVID-19 and 14 people died. COVID took the lives of 143 Saskatchewan people in February, 136 in March, and 80 in April.[36] The "mild" Omicron wave was starting to subside, but it left in its terrible wake not just death and disease but damage to the social fabric of our country.

Waving Goodbye

In the quarantine days of the pandemic, Peloton exercise bikes were selling like mad.[1] The company couldn't keep up with the demand as people looked for ways to stay in shape while they stayed home. By early 2022, the company's stock price was crashing. The panic-bought stationary bikes were now expensive clothes racks as people looked to shed anything that reminded them of being stuck at home.[2] They were ready to move on.

And so was I. The pandemic revealed how poorly the Sask Party governs. But if the NDP were going to be able to speak to Saskatchewan people about a time beyond COVID, they needed a new voice to go with that new time. Buckley Belanger, long-time MLA for Athabasca, a constituency that covers the northwest of the province, had stepped down in the summer of 2022 to take a run at federal politics. Georgina Jolibois, the mayor of La Loche, lost the by-election to replace him in February. A few days later, I announced I was stepping down as leader of the Saskatchewan NDP.

I'd been elected leader of the Opposition only four years earlier, but the pandemic years felt like they should count at least double. In a province where the government resisted meaningful action to protect public health in every wave, someone had to say the hard things. As a doctor in politics, elected on a promise to put people first, I had no choice but to be on the side of health. My team and I had to be the ones calling for things like cancelling the Junos, mandating masks, and bringing in gathering limits before the holidays. I'm confident we forced this government to do more than they ever would have done on their own, and can only imagine how much worse it would have been had they been left to their own devices. Still, I was now tied in people's minds to a restrictive time. Mild or not, Omicron was changing the game, and there was a shift in the way we were all thinking about COVID. Even for those who supported what I'd had to say, I was now a sort of "Johnny Lockdown," irrevocably associated with those hard truths, with a time people were desperate to leave behind. I'd become a Peloton.

Burning Out

That's what I told reporters on the day I announced my departure. It was all true, but of course there was more to it than that. Knowing you're done is like falling in love. Or out. You can try to explain it, but you're wrong. I'd been weighing whether to stay or to go for a long time. I'd known I had to stay through the worst of COVID. Just as there was no way I could ignore the call to return to clinical work, there was no way I could walk away while we were shipping ICU patients halfway across the country.

Still, I was exhausted. The drama within the party had grown increasingly toxic and taxing. My family wanted me home. I'd lost the taste for the "normal" politics that were about to return, working the room at another stakeholder banquet, after being on the frontline of something so all-consuming and meaningful as directly fighting for public health in the middle of a global pandemic. I wrestled, then as now, with whether it was cowardly to quit, but there came a moment when it was clear as day. The by-election gave me the clean break I needed to call it.

The sound of a bottle of pills hitting the bottom of the garbage can in my room at the Northern Sunset motel in Île-à-la-Crosse was music to my ears the morning after the Athabasca by-election. A few weeks earlier, I'd been started on an SSRI (selective serotonin reuptake inhibitor, a class of antidepressant medications) by my family doctor. It was a time of depression and confusion for people around the world, and I was no different. I've had down times in my life, but I'd never been treated for depression before. Like a lot of docs, it was hard for me to accept the help; I'm the one who cares for others, after all. I see myself as an optimist, as someone positive and joyful. At the same time, I could observe all the symptoms. My thoughts were not my own. I'd lost my enjoyment and motivation. I was waking at three or four in the morning to stir and stew, arguments and resentments spinning in my mind. I was distracted, distant, and irritable with the people I love. I wasn't myself. If a patient came to me with the same story, I'd be offering them medications as well. Depression and anxiety are serious illnesses and treating them with medications is often exactly the right thing to do. But that morning I realized I had a choice. I could keep punishing myself, keep taking pills to try to wring every last bit of serotonin from my burntout brain, or I could walk away from the pain.

I received a Facebook message from a supporter the day I announced I was stepping down. He wrote, "You did no harm." I don't know if that's true, but it brought a tear to my eye. My time in politics was a continuation of my time in medicine, and the opposite will be true as well. I'm at peace with my choice to move on. That doesn't mean it was easy. I didn't get elected with the desire to make small changes, hadn't come to fight and lose. I think about the ways I failed to bring our team together. I think of the mistakes I made in managing people and issues, sometimes too lenient or cautious, sometimes too tough or too bold. In retrospect, I think more of the errors were in going along with the tendency of progressive parties to make ourselves boring, to find loopholes to principled arguments in hopes that people will just get tired of our opponents rather than taking a stand and offering a clear alternative. Nonetheless, I believe you can be proud of who you are and what you've done but also embrace disappointment and regret. They are the burning stone of human relations; fear of them and the pull of love and joy are the lines that keep us moving straight ahead.

I was not the only one who knew it was time for a change. Kevin Wasko is an emergency medicine doctor who served on the Executive Leadership Team of the Saskatchewan Health Authority and as one of the province's pandemic leads. He is from Eastend, Saskatchewan, a small town near Swift Current where he completed his family medicine residency and later trained a new generation of rural family doctors. Dr. Wasko announced he would be leaving Saskatchewan for Ontario that February. He cited fatigue and frustration as the major factors behind his choice to move his family and his practice away from home. He has since gone on to become chief of emergency medicine at North York Hospital in Toronto.

"I am tired," he said. "I know that my colleagues, who are system leaders across the country – but here in Saskatchewan, definitely – they're tired too."[3] That fatigue comes from the clinical and administrative work itself. It also comes from watching choices being made that make things worse – understandably by the general public and much more maddeningly by those elected to lead and serve. "It is frustrating to see, amongst the public, a growing sentiment that they don't support the measures and protections that are put in place to protect our healthcare system."[4] Wasko found it increasingly disheartening to see the advice from health leadership ignored by the people with the power to make a difference. "You make the best recommendations that you can and you try to predict what could happen. It's frustrating to see when those scenarios actually play out because a decision was made to go one way or another." Kevin didn't want to stop caring, and that's why he had to walk away for a while. "I just need to take a step back for a while from that to be able to reset ... and get back some of that real joy from work that I want to have."[5]

Burnout in leadership and health care is a chronic issue that was greatly exacerbated by the pandemic. Over half of Canadian doctors reported experiencing burnout in the latest Canadian Medical Association survey, nearly twice the pre-pandemic levels.[6] When people burn out, they become emotionally exhausted, dissatisfied, and detached. They are less able to respond with compassion in their work and home lives and can wind up with full-blown depression. Newly graduated ER nurse Jacelyn Wingerter told *Maclean's*, "I love my job and my co-workers, but I leave every shift feeling incredibly upset at the state of our health care system. Every single staff member is stretched to their limits. In the last two years, many nurses, including myself, have started taking antidepressants."[7] Hailed as "health care heroes" in the early days, health care workers have put in incredibly long hours despite a diminishing level of respect from the public and decision-makers. Overtime hours for Saskatchewan nurses increased by an astonishing 4,000 percent in the first year of the pandemic.[8] Verbal and even physical abuse from patients has become commonplace, and worsened in the fourth wave as people's beliefs met the cold reality of a COVID admission.

On top of burnout, health professionals have started talking more about moral distress and moral injury. Moral injury is what happens when system constraints make it impossible to make the ethical choice, creating a situation where people are forced to "do, witness, or are unable to prevent, something that goes against their strongly held values and beliefs."[9] The most striking example is that of "ethical triage," where doctors have been put in the position of deciding who gets care and who is denied, even who lives and who dies, because the choices weren't made that could protect their ability to provide care. There are many more: long-term care workers forced to deny family visitation, hospital staff having to decide whether their exposure was risky enough to leave their co-workers understaffed, frontline witnesses of the effects of political choices agonizing over whether they should speak up or whether it will do any good if they do. The constant moral distress is one more source of exhaustion and depression that has people questioning whether they can continue to care.

As a result, more and more health care professionals are considering decreasing their practice or walking away from the profession entirely. Two-thirds of doctors surveyed by the Saskatchewan Medical Association reported that their mental health had worsened over the course of the pandemic.[10] The majority said they would be reducing their hours of service in the next two years, and one in five were considering retiring in that time. The "lack of physician voice in the pandemic response" was a major source of frustration for three-quarters of respondents. Registered nurses responding to a Saskatchewan Union of Nurses survey described chronic short-staffing, and over half reported they were considering leaving the profession entirely.[11] When people lose the emotional connection to the work they used to love, it becomes easier to walk away, to seek out work that pays more or has less responsibility, rather than going where their service is most needed. As Saskatchewan Medical Association president Eben Strydom pointed out, this poses a major risk: "At this stage, we need ... healthy physicians. We need energized physicians. We need all hands to deal with the challenges ahead."[12] Failing to recognize and respond to health care worker burnout is a recipe for more burnout, more moral injury, and worse care for Canadians who need it.

While I'd made my decision and announcement to leave as leader, I had one more legislative session ahead. Two people had come forward to run for the leadership, Saskatoon lawyer Kaitlyn Harvey and Regina MLA Carla Beck. All signs pointed to the membership supporting Carla, but of course I stayed neutral on that question. My focus was on having a successful session and handing over the reins in the most helpful way I could. Scott Moe gave us some help with that. When he was asked about carbon emissions at an April 2022 Prince Albert Chamber of Commerce event, he replied, "I don't care."[13] These are not great words for a politician to use at any time, but with his record from the last two years it was impossible not to extrapolate from climate change to health care to unemployment – you name it. This gave us a new way to talk about all the growing troubles under his leadership, and for me to maintain focus on the government's record.

First Response

After the provincial budget is presented, each ministry has what are called "estimates," where their budgets are afforded a certain number of hours of direct scrutiny. The critics for each ministry have the opportunity to directly question the ministers and the officials from their departments. This doesn't get the attention that question period does, but instead of pointed questions and deflective answers, it's often where we learn about real issues.

The last of these sessions is referred to as "Premier's Estimates." This is a lot more like question period, but instead of the usual twenty-five minutes, the leader of the Opposition questions the premier for three straight hours. Though mired by long pauses and rambling self-congratulatory asides – I often likened debating Scott Moe to punching a marshmallow – there are moments of heated debate and the occasional memorable exchange. It's also the one set of estimates that the media watches closely, so I always spent extra time preparing.

One evening I decided to go for supper and work on my questions. I walked from my downtown apartment to Korea House on 11th Street.

This is one of my favourite spots in Regina, a neighbourhood with character and lots of different international restaurants and shops. A little further down is Pepsi Park, where a tent city had popped up for a few weeks the previous fall. At the time there were about seventy tents with over a hundred people living in the park as winter approached. Many found themselves homeless after a change in social services programming left people without the supports to pay the rent. The camp was originally referred to as Camp Marjorie, after someone who had died while homeless. It was later renamed Camp Hope, and an incredible effort was made by the residents of the park and community organizations supporting them to provide meals and warm blankets and to work toward a safer indoor space.

A good plate of bibimbap and a few pages of notes later, I walked out the front door of Korea House in a bit of a writing fog. I snapped out of it when I saw someone in a white hoodie collapsing in the bus shelter across the street. Two people were calling his name and trying to stand him up but he kept sliding to the ground. "Did he overdose?" I asked the two men and a woman standing there. One guy with longer white hair asked if I had Narcan. I said no and asked him to run to the pharmacy two blocks away. I examined the young man. He still had a strong pulse but was not responsive to sternal rub and not visibly breathing. A woman about my age with purplish hair had 911 on the phone. They said Fire was on the way and asked me to watch his breathing.

Suddenly the young man who had overdosed gave one big, deep breath and then nothing for thirty seconds. His pulse started to become fainter. I was worried he might die right then and there. I started chest compressions with the 911 operator counting them off on speakerphone. That coaching wasn't really necessary, but it was nice to be connected to someone whose presence meant that help was on its way. After a few compressions, he perked up for a second, opened his eyes, gasped, then collapsed again. I took that chance to check his pulse. Much stronger now. I kept going with compressions for three or four more counts of thirty.

A fire truck pulled up and a crew of EMTs jumped out. Within moments they had a bag-valve-mask going to help him breathe and a shot of naloxone in his shoulder to counteract the effects of the opioid drugs. I stepped back and watched for a while as they established a blood pressure and it was clear he was past the worst. As usual, when you're the first responder before the first responder, no one pays you much attention. I did the awkward thing of standing around, knowing I couldn't be of more help but feeling like I should, like a medical student on rounds. Eventually, one of the EMTs asked me to give them some room in the shelter and I moved back.

I asked the woman and the other guy, a short man with a ball cap, if they knew the young man. The woman had just been driving by when she saw him lying down in the shelter and pulled around. The other guy was walking with his friend and they saw him down as well. He thought it was someone he'd been in treatment with a few years back, but the name he called him by turned out not to be his right name. I then put my hand on the woman's shoulder and told her, "I think you saved his life." And it's true, she had. I told the guy with the ball cap the same thing and started my walk back to the apartment.

As I passed by the Al Madina halal grocery store, a pre-teen kid walked out, cracked a two-litre bottle of root beer, and took a swig. He looked down the street and turned to his friend to say, blasé as can be, "Somebody overdosed." It was an intense event for those directly involved, but in the neighbourhood it had become ordinary, an everyday occurrence. And with nearly 450 overdoses in Saskatchewan the year before, every day is an understatement. During the time the camp was in Pepsi Park, one person died of an overdose in their tent.[14] After it was shut down, at least nine more of those who had been staying there would die by spring.[15]

The sun was setting as I walked home thinking about what had happened in that bus shelter. We were just down the street from Regina's only safe consumption site, but it doesn't have funding to open in the evenings. If those good Samaritans who had shown up and called 911 hadn't been there, it was a matter of minutes before that young man's life would have been over forever. Another person to add to the 327 Saskatchewan people who lost their lives to overdose in 2020, 410 in 2021, and 421 in 2022, another unbelievably tragic record.[16] I thought about Cory Cardinal, about parents like Marie Agioritis of Moms Stop the Harm grieving the unbelievable loss of their child, about the patients I'd counselled and sought care for only to learn they were never coming back.

And for every person who dies, how many more had a near-miss? How many more are alive but in desperate circumstances and destroying their lives with drugs? How many are wondering where they'll spend the night? As I walked home, I got angry again just thinking about the social services program changes that left more people homeless, the lack of access to in-patient addictions care, or the decision to not fund safe consumption sites. Different choices for every one of those decisions might have prevented that young man's situation. Every decision to not help sends people in trouble the message that they're just not worth it.

I reflected on my own minor role in responding to that overdose. I'd been advocating for years for harm reduction policy, knowing it wasn't what political people call a "vote-getter." On that night, I'd been in the right place at the right time and had some dormant skills that may have contributed to keeping that young man alive. I was also reminded that, at the end of the day, I was a doctor in politics. It's why I was there, it's why I cared. Having the reputation and the instincts of a doctor was the source of some of my successes and some of my failures. And as I was walking off into the sunset of my career in provincial politics, I wondered what I might have learned that I would carry with me back into clinical practice, what good and bad habits I would bring as a recovering politician in medicine.

The House Rises

Gus and I stopped in front of the statue of Tommy Douglas in the rotunda at the legislature on my last day. I told him who Tommy was, trying to explain in terms a four-year-old could understand what the legislature was about and why Medicare was so important. Gus was born during the 2018 leadership race; he'd never known me outside politics. His dad working in this weird castle in Regina was just normal. I tried to tell him why that building mattered, why it had been such an honour to be able to hold an office that had seen the likes of Tommy, Woodrow Lloyd, Allan Blakeney, Roy Romanow, and Lorne Calvert. He humoured me for a bit, then ran off to play with his brother.

Mahli, Abe, and Gus were there, along with my parents, my brother Jim, and friends from my political and personal life. After the usual question period, Carla Beck moved a motion of thanks as a farewell. She, the premier, and MLAs on our side made some very gracious comments. I responded with my final speech, a few anecdotes, and the requisite number of corny jokes, a sincere apology for the times I'd lost my cool or let things get too personal, and a lot of thank-yous. And just as I'd tried to tell Gus on our way in that day, I spoke of what it means to stand in the people's house. From the first nervous moment through hundreds of question period questions, introductions of guests, presenting and receiving petitions, and statements by members, things become routine. Yet every time, when you take to your feet to make a speech there's a lump in your throat. Because the legislature does matter.

Each of us plays for a season or two, but long after we're gone, what we say on the record will stand. The building will still stand long after everybody who was in it that day has been laid to rest. And the work of democracy will go on long after we walk away. It matters for history, for understanding how today is built on yesterday and how tomorrow will make its home atop today. It also matters because of what those words can do, how they can change the circumstances of real people for better or worse, for what they can change and for what they can preserve and protect. They matter for the difference that they make. Like everyone there, I had come hoping to make a difference.

People speak about the sacrifice of political life, and certainly there was some. But the rewards, the joys of the job, were incredible. I saw the province in ways few get the chance to, from places like Fond du Lac in the Far North to visiting drought-stricken ranches on the US border. I shared in the grief of families who lost a child or the joy of a community opening a new school just as in medicine we share the sorrows of illness and death and the joys of cures and new birth.

Every person matters as much as anyone else, and we all do better when we remember that we're all in this together. That's my core belief and what I see as the core belief of the social democratic movement. I also see that idea in Paul Farmer's favourite Haitian Creole proverb, *tout moun se moun,* which translates to "every person is a person." Farmer was an infectious disease specialist, an anthropologist, and co-founder of the international medical NGO Partners In Health (PIH). PIH articulates the principle as "All human lives have the same value, and every human being has the inalienable right to be healthy to fulfill their potential."[17]

I've been thinking a lot about Farmer since he died suddenly in Rwanda in 2021 at the age of sixty-two. No contemporary physician can compare with the influence Paul Farmer has had on a generation of doctors. In his seminal 2003 book, *Pathologies of Power*, he wrote: "It took me a relatively short time in Haiti to discover that I could never serve as a dispassionate reporter or chronicler of misery. I am only on the side of the destitute sick and have never sought to represent myself as some sort of neutral party."[18] Reading his articulation of structural violence in Haiti and Peru helped give me the vocabulary to describe what I was seeing in Mozambique or inner-city Saskatoon. His writing on the connection between liberation theology and social medicine spoke directly to my reasons for becoming a doctor.

Farmer used to speak of the "long defeat" of siding with those whose lives are stacked against them. This is inherent in the kind of medicine he practised, a preferential option for the poor against the crushing inequities within countries and between the poorest countries and the wealthiest. He won a lot – his work and the work of PIH have saved millions of lives – but it was still the long defeat. To extend the analogy, it's a concept inherent to medicine as well: no matter how good your treatment, all of your patients will die. As Dr. Rieux admitted in *The Plague*, all our victories against illness and death are temporary, "but that is not a reason to give up the struggle."[19]

Farmer was never a politician, but his work and writing were deeply political. Politics, too, is a game of the long defeat. Win or lose elections, the change you hope to make will always be receding. For me, the experience of elected life was all a part of the long defeat, and believing that, because the lives of human beings matter, it's still worth fighting for every win you can even when the ultimate outcome is certain.

It's bittersweet. The work is bittersweet and so is its end. It's good to know when you're done; it feels right, but there is still grief. The biggest disappointment is the loss of "someday." When you're first getting involved in politics and someone brings you something hard, something that isn't working for them, you try to help them in the moment.

At the same time, you tell yourself, someday we'll be in government, someday we'll fix this. You look around and see the injustice, the unfairness of the world, and you think, it doesn't have to be this way and I'm going to do something about it. That's what keeps people going through the hard days of campaigning and debating, of every action being subject to scrutiny and judgment. The someday makes it worthwhile. Saying goodbye to that is hard.

But do you know what else is bittersweet? Lemonade. And I've always had a great recipe for lemonade. I have had a chance to live such great adventures in medicine and politics. I don't know where life will lead me next, but I know I'll keep working for health and that this experience will inform the next steps in ways I can't yet imagine. The pandemic isn't done with us, politics isn't done with us. Years from now we will look around and say, "We're doing things this way because of what we learned in the early 2020s." There's no way to tell for sure until we're there, but by taking stock of what has happened and identifying some key lessons, we can set ourselves up to learn and make the most of what we've all been through.

Lessons for the Next Wave

From the first whispers of a new virus, through quarantine and vaccines, and on to Omicron and long COVID, our experience of the pandemic has shifted. Approaches that were obvious at the beginning were discarded by the second wave. Policies necessary to get us through the worst times have had unintended consequences. Imperfect messaging led to long-lasting misconceptions and resentments. As destructive as this crisis has been, it can also be instructive, provided we don't succumb to the all-too-human temptation to just put it all behind us. We all want to return to something more normal, but it would be a tremendous mistake to simply go back to the way things were. The way things were wasn't working. If COVID revealed what was broken, can it also reveal how to fix it?

The COVID-19 pandemic represents the biggest disruption to every-day life most of us have ever experienced. Many people can, however, relate to times when setbacks like a difficult breakup or losing a job led to reflection and a better life. Disruption is unsettling, but it can also force us to examine how we were living before and lead to positive change. This is our moment to take a long, hard look in the mirror and ask our-selves what kind of future we want.

It's natural to want the mirror in question to be a rear-view one. It's also crucial that we don't pretend we're further along than we are. Canada saw more COVID deaths in 2022 than in either of the two previous years, and the same is true for Saskatchewan.[1] It may be too soon to move on completely, but it's by no means too soon to start learning the lessons from this experience.

During the height of COVID, I was often asked what I thought was going to happen next. Would the vaccines work? Would we get new versions of the virus? Would this last for years or was this latest wave finally the end? My answer was always the same: the smartest people in the world have no idea. The degrees of how educated the guesses are vary, but everyone is guessing. Predicting the future is a mug's game. Preparing for a variety of possible futures by learning from the experiences of the recent past is a lot more useful.

One thing that's obvious is that the pace of life pre-pandemic is optional. We don't have to live as fast and blind as we have. We can stop, take a deep breath, and ask what kind of country we want to live in. What is our vision for our home and for our world? What can we learn and what can we become?

1. The best measure of a society is the health of its people

Since the onset of COVID-19, people have thought about health in a way we never have before. At the peak of the pandemic, daily case counts, hospitalizations, and deaths were water cooler conversation. Epidemiological concepts of positivity rates, herd immunity, and community transmission were understood and discussed by people who'd never had a moment's interest in public health.

Whether it was the Atlantic Bubble compared with the Prairies, the exemplary record of New Zealand, or the disaster of Peru, the relative success of jurisdictions was measured by health outcomes. From this moment of great intensity comes a longer-term principle. The best measure of a society's success at any time is the health of its people. Just as all of our dreams, interests, and ambitions quickly fade in importance when we're faced with our own illness or that of someone close to us, how long your citizens live, their "physical, social and mental well-being,"[2] these are the things that matter most. Economic success is an enormous contributor to that goal, but it's not the goal itself. With health identified as our primary objective, we can then turn our attention to what will make a difference in improving health.

One way to turn that idea into action is with the concept of Health in All Policies, an approach that "systematically takes into account the health and health systems implications of decisions, seeks synergies and avoids harmful health impacts, in order to improve population health and health equity."[3] It's not just the Ministry of Health that determines the health of the population. Decisions made in every part of government – finance, justice, environment, education, you name it – have a profound influence on people's health. With optimal health as our destination, the social determinants of health provide the roadmap to do the most good. COVID has shown us where we need to act by highlighting the problems in work, in schools, in health care, and in elder care. Incorporating a "whole-of-government" approach can turn that understanding into real results.

Throughout the pandemic, and especially in the earliest days, we saw how government can be a tremendous force for good. Practically overnight, there were not only sweeping public health measures but also massive investments to meet the pressing economic and social needs of the population. Governments matter. Those who argue for smaller, less effective government on principle are arguing that we should be less ready for major challenges. There is nothing inherently good in smaller or larger government; it's about having the public capacity to intervene on behalf of people at the right level, no more and no less. A Health in All Policies approach can help determine that right level by guiding how we use the tool of government and measure the effectiveness of its use.

Achieving that new model of health-focused governance is a major change. If we want a government that truly works for us, we need to demand it over and over again. Health in All Policies can't be something we only turn on in a crisis, however. It needs to be the long-term bedrock of healthy public policy that makes the most of the good times and creates the resilience we need to make it through the bad. Changing the political discourse in such a fundamental way is a massive challenge. It won't be accomplished by this book, by any one speech, or by any single politician. To reframe the conversation to what matters most, we need a consistent political movement that demands it. Coming out of a global pandemic, where the importance of public intervention for public health was made clearer than ever before, is the perfect time for that movement to emerge.

2. A healthy economy requires healthy people

During the COVID-19 pandemic, the loop of making choices upstream to avoid future problems went from decades to days. We saw natural experiments play out as countries or regions that took starkly different approaches had vastly different rates of death and disease, and drastically different economic impacts. A fall 2020 review of the COVID response and economic performance of thirty-eight countries showed that, "among countries with available GDP data, we do not see any evidence of a trade-off between protecting people's health and protecting the economy. The relationship we see between the health and economic impacts of the pandemic goes in the opposite direction. As well as saving lives, countries controlling the outbreak effectively may have adopted the best economic strategy too."[4]

A 2021 study found that parts of Canada that adopted an elimination approach did much better than those that "emphasized impacts on the economy over the other considerations."[5] In Saskatchewan, that perceived economic trade-off led a business-first Saskatchewan Party government to err on the side of illness. "If the premier is right that major economic damage is the unacceptable price of a convincing victory over the virus, it becomes a pick-your-poison scenario: your money or your life," wrote Saskatchewan health policy experts Steven Lewis, Nazeem Muhajarine, and Cory Neudorf in a 2021 op-ed.[6] They went on to describe how analysis in the science journal *Nature* showed that the governments around the world that did as little as possible as late as possible saw much greater economic contractions than those that took early, decisive action.[7] In Canada and around the world, those who were willing to sacrifice lives for money lost both.

The idea that we had to trade people's health for the sake of the economy was wrong. The places that took better care of their humans took better care of their money as well. That's great news, because what was true at high speed in the peak of the pandemic is true in the slower pace of ordinary times as well. Investing in people, who are the heart of the economy, is the key to economic success. Healthy people go to work, start businesses, pay taxes, make art, enjoy life. If we want long-term economic success, the health of human beings is not a side benefit, it's the foundation.

In early 2020, Saskatchewan's economy was hit hard, uniquely vulnerable to the international shocks that crashed prices for commodities like oil and potash. In 2022, Russia's invasion of Ukraine sent those prices soaring, bringing massive revenues into provincial coffers, but also driving up the cost of living for ordinary people.[8] It's hard to imagine that the boom-and-bust cycle that has been a defining feature of the Prairie economy for over a century won't continue to some degree, but there are important conversations to be had about how we can be less vulnerable to the ups and downs of world events. The troubles that left grocery meat counters and new vehicle lots empty have raised questions about global supply chains and local production. In the scramble to roll out COVID vaccines, we had to face the fact that Canada had gone from a world leader in vaccine development to having zero capacity for domestic vaccine production.[9] A virus that emerged in one corner of the world and changed in another has reminded us of the strengths and vulnerabilities of our global connections.

In 2017, a group convened by the Saskatchewan Chamber of Commerce and several key industry organizations interviewed business leaders from across Saskatchewan about their views on building a more resilient provincial economy. The resulting *Upstream Economy* report placed particular emphasis on education, health, and engagement of Indigenous peoples.[10] It spoke of "the need to concentrate efforts on and direct investment in upstream transformation" as "Saskatchewan's greatest opportunity to generate growth, wealth, and an ever-improving quality of life for the next generation."[11]

Our consideration of how to build that upstream economy must consider the role of people caring for people. In 2020, a group of researchers and economists started the Care Economy Initiative, looking to redefine our understanding of spending in health and education from "costs" to "investments that stimulate the economy and safeguard our health." Pointing out that "paid care in health and education alone is a key engine of the economy, generating at least 12% of GDP and 21% of jobs," they make a strong case for the care economy as a central component to longer-term economic stability.[12] Moving our economy upstream can help us to safeguard Canada's abundant natural and human resource wealth from future shocks and maximize our opportunities to contribute to people's well-being here and around the world.

3. More equal societies are healthier, including during a pandemic

Inequality is the world's biggest killer. Patients might at first seem to be sick because of bacteria or a cancer cell, but in reality they are sick because they never had a chance at a decent education, a decent job, sick because they couldn't afford a safe place to live or healthy food for themselves and their families.

The Commission on Social Determinants of Health, led by Sir Michael Marmot, said in its landmark report *Closing the Gap in a Generation* that "social injustice is killing people on a grand scale."[13] In his work, Marmot describes the way in which inequalities, globally and within societies, lead to inequities – unfair differences – in health outcomes. While no part of the world and no social group was fully spared from COVID, we again saw those inequities play out in the scale of the impact. A Health Canada study showed higher rates of death and illness in communities of lower socio-economic status, among visible minorities, and among those who speak neither official language.[14] A study by Public Health Montreal revealed that not only were death rates in poorer areas of the city more than double those in the wealthier neighbourhoods but each quintile of difference in income was associated with a significant difference in outcomes with the group above or below.[15]

Internationally, differences in equality appear to have a significant influence on COVID outcomes between countries. This analysis was partly spurred by observations that outcomes were not as strongly linked with heavier public health restrictions as expected. *The Economist* reported that, "faced with these surprising results, a hunt has begun that is as morbid as it is nerdy. Wonks are searching for less obvious variables that do more to explain variation in deaths from COVID-19. And so far the most powerful of them all is inequality – usually measured as the Gini coefficient of income, where zero represents perfect equality and one represents perfect inequality."[16] Inequality was the largest correlating factor for different outcomes between US states,[17] and a McGill University study looking at eighty-four countries found that a 1 percent increase in equality was associated with a 0.67 percent decrease in COVID mortality.[18] The more equal the country or state, the better it did through COVID-19. This is consistent with the research of Richard Wilkinson and Kate Pickett as described in their seminal work, *The Spirit Level:* the more unequal a society, the worse the health outcomes at every level, not just for those most disadvantaged.[19] People who live in more unequal societies have worse health in general. People who are poor and excluded in any society experience more sickness and die earlier. Martin Luther King Jr. said that "of all the forms of inequality, injustice in health is the most shocking and inhumane."[20] Aside from being unfair to those who suffer the illness, these inequities also impose an enormous burden of added cost in Canada and around the world.

Marmot's Institute of Health Equity lays out the need to put equity at the centre of our pandemic response in its COVID-19 review, *Build Back Fairer:*

> There is an urgent need to do things differently, to build a society based on the principles of social justice; to reduce inequalities of income and wealth; to build a well-being economy that puts achievement of health and well-being at the heart of government strategy, rather than narrow economic goals; to build a society that responds to the climate crisis at the same time as achieving greater health equity.[21]

If we want a healthier future for Canada, addressing inequality at every level must be central to that effort. This means working to assist the most vulnerable in society: those without stable housing, the people who find themselves in a prison system structured to perpetuate crime and addiction, those who are excluded due to race, language, or religion, the very young and the very old.

4. Facts are worth fighting for

In many ways, the story of COVID is one of both a communicable disease and a communication disease. Or, in the words of World Health

Organization director-general Dr. Tedros Adhanom Ghebreyesus: "We're not just fighting an epidemic; we're fighting an infodemic. Fake news spreads faster and more easily than this coronavirus and is just as dangerous."[22] We were told to reduce our contacts and stay in our bubbles. Social media already had us there. The decline of traditional media means that sources of information more subject to scrutiny of their quality and veracity have given way to the unaccountable fever swamps of specialized rage-farming sites, YouTube rabbit holes, and the toxic trolling of Facebook feeds, Twitter replies, and comment sections. If misinformation was a smouldering fire, COVID was a steady stream of gasoline.

Twila Lamont was a thirty-six-year-old mother of six from Yorkton. When COVID hit her household in November 2021, she and her husband, Derek Langan, decided they should ride it out at home because the hospitals were full. The Saskatchewan Health Authority had stopped their previous practice of daily calls to check up on identified positives. Had they been calling, they might have learned that things were going very badly. Derek hardly left his bed for two weeks and wasn't aware of how ill his wife was. She was found unresponsive. Despite being barely able to walk, Derek attempted CPR, but it was too late for Twila. Derek later told the CBC that they decided not to get vaccinated because of things they'd read on Facebook, stories he now sees as "myths and conspiracy theories."[23]

These same Facebook myths and conspiracy theories are now informing the actions of governments. Disingenuous politicians fed into this from early days, with then US president Donald Trump a primary culprit. Dissenting scientific voices were given platforms on popular podcasts and propaganda news channels, not because their views were well examined and found credible but because they were dissenting. Reputations that should have been damaged by repeating falsehoods were instead enhanced and fringe falsehoods became mainstream messages. As Stephen Maher pointed out, writing in *Maclean's*, "there are three times as many COVID deaths in Trump-supporting counties, where vaccination rates are low, as there are in Democratic counties. In Canada, the areas most heavily influenced by Trump-style politics are also the areas with the highest rates of vaccine resistance."[24] Just as resonating vibrations can destroy a bridge, the exponential spread of lies without consequence is a threat not only to public health in a pandemic but to the institutions that form the foundation of a nation.

Combatting disinformation is now central to the project of maintaining liberal democracy and public health. We ignore poisonous resistance at our peril, but caving to it is not the answer. What is the role of the social media giants in policing the veracity of what is shared on their platforms? How do parliaments and legislatures promote facts and discourage falsehoods? How can civil society and scholars compete in the clickbait marketplace with those unfettered by ethics?

The immediate crisis of a rapidly emerging and changing pandemic laid bare the challenge of communicating complex issues in the face of deliberate disinformation. Too many people are unwilling to change until it's too late, even when too late is in two weeks. We've learned the hard way that we must plan ahead and prepare for the worst, no matter how hard making decisions for tomorrow may be. We also learned how hard it is to bring people into that planning. It is daunting to think how we will be able to ask people to make major changes and sacrifices for something as large and nebulous as climate change when sustaining minor inconveniences in the face of imminent danger was too much to ask.

In the face of mounting disinformation, we will need stronger voices for evidence-based solutions. We saw increased advocacy from many sectors and professions during the pandemic. Some of these voices were extremely effective and drove change; others got caught up in the same cycle of likes and retweets that drives their opponents, becoming more extreme in their positions and undermining their own credibility. Academic institutions and governments can work together to study what kinds of evidence-based advocacy work and amplify credible sources. We need to help people with knowledge and understanding to say the hard things and have them heard, to spread neither doom and gloom nor false hope, but a vision of the best future we can build together.

5. We need to trust people with the truth, even as the truth changes

Our scientific and public understanding of the virus has grown dramatically and quickly. The change can be tracked with the changes in our vocabulary, from "novel coronavirus" to familiarity with subsets of various variants, from "surface transmission" to "hygiene theatre." When we say to follow the science, inherent in that idea is that our scientific understanding develops and we must be able to adapt to new knowledge. The great risk lies in insisting that what we know at one point is what we will always know and refusing to change earlier assumptions as we learn more. In the dance of the pandemic, the science leads. The steps change; we have to learn to follow.

Much as a patient might move from a hyperglycemic emergency to adjusting to the reality of living with diabetes, we have moved with COVID from immediate response to medium-term mitigation and long-term adaptation. Daily inconveniences, like testing sugars or keeping a box of masks in the car for when they are needed, become substantial changes that reflect what we've learned about how to stay healthy, be they constant diet and lifestyle demands on the personal level or new approaches to public policy at the societal level. The right choices change and the challenges of communicating them become more complex.

Downplaying the seriousness of the situation and restricting the data erode public trust in official channels. As André Picard noted in a March 2022 *Globe and Mail* column, "throughout the pandemic we have consistently looked for ways to downplay its severity, from claiming older people felled by COVID-19 were going to die anyhow, to distinguishing people hospitalized 'from' COVID-19 from those 'with' COVID-19."[25] Despite having some of the world's most sophisticated and accurate modelling, what was seen by the Saskatchewan public was largely the result of leaks or freedom of information requests rather than proactive sharing of information. When it was shared, "best case scenarios" were emphasized without the acknowledgment that these could only be achieved with significant change. "Road maps" for coming choices were either absent or solely focused on how to respond if things got better, not what to do if they got worse. We had a chance to let people see the facts and invite them into a conversation about how to shape the days ahead, and we blew it in favour of brightsiding. When we acknowledge problems and mistakes honestly, people are willing to engage. When everything is about damage control and spin, people walk away.

That's why trusting people with the truth and demonstrating that trust through transparency is so crucial. Knowing how many cases there were, where they were located, where deaths were occurring – this is the kind of information that helps people understand their risk and make wise choices. Knowing the next steps if things worsen or improve gives people agency. When people feel trusted, they are more likely to trust. When information is kept from people, that's when suspicion creeps in, leaving people uncertain about how to act or even susceptible to the types of conspiracy theories that are flourishing today.

Part of trusting people includes telling them not just what you know but what you don't. In the earliest days of the pandemic, we were shunning masks and disinfecting our groceries. Later, vaccines were going to end things once and for all. Again from Picard: "If there is one overarching lesson from the pandemic, it is that messaging matters. And the messages need to be nuanced. We need a lot less black-and-white, and a lot more grey." Not only do we need to share with people the information we do have, we also need to be honest about what we don't know. When we let people know in advance that things will change, it allows the space for our understanding and messaging to evolve. If you set people up to think things are simple, straightforward, and once and for all, they will be frustrated when they aren't.

Despite the Omicron wave being among the deadliest in our pandemic experience, most people remember it as the end, because that's when we stopped receiving daily updates on cases, hospitalizations, and deaths. Stretching these updates out to weekly and later monthly took away the means to stay engaged. It may not have worked to reduce the transmission of the virus, but it was tremendously successful in reducing the attention being paid to it. Rather than learning the lesson that greater transparency will improve the public response to challenging times, I worry some leaders will decide that it's to their benefit to stop sharing information sooner. For example, in response to growing concern in the fall of 2022 that there were no family physicians taking new patients in Regina or Saskatoon, the public posting of that information was discontinued.[26]

Telling people less in order to decrease criticism is not the path to a healthier, more open society. Responsible leaders who genuinely want to combat misinformation need to make information as widely available and accessible as possible. It's not a matter of simply telling people to trust in the experts; that sort of technocratic response will not work in a democratic society. The decisions on how to build a healthier future need to be in the hands of the people. This leaves a challenge in the hands of the politically engaged public: exercising our democratic rights includes demanding all the facts. We need to insist that governments trust us with the truth.

6. Leaders need to learn to work together in times of crisis

After an initial period of being "all in this together," the level of distrust and polarization between people of opposing views has grown through the pandemic. In those early days, we had an opportunity to set the stage for cross-party collaboration. It may have been difficult to achieve or maintain – with the pending snap election the animosity between the political players was already high – but it was worth a try. There are examples of where this was done, both historical and recent. Collaboration between federal, municipal, and provincial agencies made a massively successful vaccine rollout possible.

Going forward, leaders from across the political spectrum must look for opportunities to invite people in to help in moments of crisis. The current agreement between federal Liberals and New Democrats, while panned among those who disapprove of our current prime minister, may be a good example of parties finding a way to put aside differences to achieve shared goals in challenging times. Was there a possibility of inviting federal Conservatives to be part of a more constructive conversation on COVID at the beginning of the pandemic? Might that have created some degree of check on the later tendency of Canada's right wing to follow the more extreme rhetoric coming from Trump Republicans? Perhaps the outcomes would have been the same, perhaps those forces of division and disinformation are too hard to resist, but isn't trying even when it's difficult what leadership is about?

In times of crisis, the need for collaboration is manifestly present. The cool heads needed to do it well may not be. Working together civilly and effectively is a muscle that requires training. Governments and oppositions across Canada should be seeking ways to build up that collaborative capacity in regular times so that, in the event of another emergency, it is easier to find the space to work together. One might even propose the establishment of a legislative secretary or other official position to facilitate cross-party collaboration and normalize non-adversarial experiences between members of different parties, rather than have their only interactions be in the heat of the assembly or the refreshments line at a reception.

7. For Medicare to work, we need to build a robust and resilient health system

"Health systems were never designed for this kind of surge. I think federal governments for decades have been underfunding things like public health preparedness."[27] This is what then federal health minister Patty Hajdu had to say in April 2020 when questioned about Canada's readiness for the pandemic. A 2006 pandemic preparedness report coauthored by now chief public health officer of Canada Theresa Tam had suffered the fate of many such reports, its recommendations gathering dust as people moved on from the 2003 SARS epidemic.[28] The owner of a dumpster bin company in Regina broke the story of the federal government's disposal of two million N95 masks and 440,000 medical gloves in 2019 without replenishing the stockpile.[29] In March 2021 Canada's auditor general released a scathing review of the Public Health Agency of Canada's preparation: "The agency was not adequately prepared to respond to the pandemic, and it underestimated the potential impact of the virus at the onset of the pandemic."[30]

Ontario premier Doug Ford cut $200 million from public health agencies in his province in 2019.[31] Two months after the first cases of COVID-19 had arrived in Canada, we learned in question period that not a single additional dollar had been dedicated to public health in Saskatchewan.[32] Cuts to public health are often buried in global budgets and thus difficult to delineate, but spending in prevention and health promotion is frequently first on the chopping block when competing for funding against clinical care. Failing to plan for the future is beyond unwise.

This applies beyond the field of public health to the provision of health care overall. Governments have been "redlining" their health care systems, running them at or slightly beyond capacity at all times. This manifests in chronic understaffing in acute and long-term care settings, staff burnout and turnover, and an inability to respond to added pressures when they arrive. In Saskatchewan, this was taken to extremes with the 2008 introduction of the "Lean" program, an ill-fated attempt at hyper-efficiency based on Toyota's production line philosophy. One peer-reviewed evaluation of this experiment found the cost of contracts for its implementation to be far higher than any savings, with no improvement in patient outcomes and a significant decrease in job satisfaction among nurses.[33]

The current nationwide health care crisis – with shortages of family doctors and nursing staff, overflowing emergency rooms and pediatric wards, and long wait times for imaging and surgery – is the long tail effect of a major stress event on an already overstretched system. It is an acute-on-chronic problem with no easy solutions. There are, however, some principles that can help us plot our way to the other side and rebuild a health care system that works for people:

- *Public care is the best care.* We need to resist the temptation – and the efforts of those who would profit from this crisis – to throw up our hands and let the forces of privatization take over. The dismal record of the for-profit sector in protecting long-term care residents should be enough to kill that idea, but free market absolutist ideologues wait eagerly in the wings to take advantage of this moment. We should not only fight to keep what is within Medicare public but also keep our eye on the larger cost savings and improvements in outcomes associated with expansions into areas such as Pharmacare. A major area of focus needs to be increased access to primary care, including concentrated efforts to address the nationwide shortage of family physicians. High-quality primary care gives patients comprehensive attention while they're still well, catching illness earlier, improving patient outcomes, and reducing pressures on our emergency rooms and in-patient wards.

- *The system needs slack.* We have tried running a health system with just enough or not-quite-enough capacity. It doesn't work for patients, it doesn't work for providers, and it certainly doesn't work for pandemics. As I wrote this chapter, Mahli was on call and the pediatric department was beyond swamped. Every in-patient bed was full, every emergency room bed was full, and there were dozens of kids in the waiting room. This had a lot to do with the "triple-demic" wave of RSV, influenza, and COVID rocking the lungs of Canadian kids at the time, but it isn't an isolated event. It has more to do with the fact that the province built a brand-new, shiny children's hospital in 2019 that had fewer in-patient beds than the old Royal University Hospital pediatric ward it replaced. When you build a bookshelf, you shouldn't build it for the books you already have.

  Whether it's short-staffing in long-term care, rural emergency rooms that can't stay open, or the lack of mental health and addictions beds, we have undershot capacity for years. It's time to go in the other direction. It's time to create good jobs in the care economy, an investment in people that pays back. It's time for us to train, credential, and hire more people than we think we need. I'm not talking about having people sit around and be paid to do nothing. I'm talking about not having people run off their feet every shift, about not burning out everyone we have and being unable to recruit anyone new because the dream of the caring professions has become a waking nightmare.

  Public health is a good place to start. Testing and contact tracing for infectious diseases, for example, is a place where "excess capacity" can be well-applied to control endemic diseases like syphilis, gonorrhea, tuberculosis, and HIV, all of which have seen significant spikes in Saskatchewan during COVID. Added capacity allows for more research and quality improvement, more promotion of evidence-based information on immunization to combat growing anti-vax disinformation, and more time to work upstream, addressing the social determinants of health. In acute and long-term care, ending the constant experience of working short-handed will allow for greater collegiality, higher retention, and better patient and resident experiences and outcomes. By "overstaffing" in health – and in other crucial areas such as education – we can build the kind of robust and resilient public system that goes above and beyond for the well-being of Canadians in ordinary times and is prepared to tackle the unprecedented.

8. To learn the lessons, our stories must be shared

In November 2022, one year after the Saskatchewan organ donation program was suspended, Jessica Bailey finally got the help she needed. Despite losing her first donor, despite her health getting so bad she was considered palliative, she didn't give up. And her doctors didn't give up on her either. With their help, she was able to get her blood pressure under control and be fit enough to receive a transplant. Her sister was also able to improve her own health enough that she could be Jessica's donor. I spoke to Jessica that December and she told me her new kidney was the best Christmas present she'd ever had. A story that had come so close to avoidable and unnecessary tragedy had taken a hopeful turn.

Jessica, Fred Sasakamoose, Alice Grove, Matty Cardinal, Dr. Palangi, Helen Dickson, Ken Roth – there is a reason I share their stories. Partly it's because it's easier for us to connect to ideas when we meet them in the shape of real people. More importantly, it's because I've seen how quickly numbers cease to mean much of anything at all. As the pandemic wore on, even as the case counts and death totals rose, the level of public concern and political action fell. The stories were lost in the statistics.

"Remember Rebuild Saskatchewan" is a project of the University of Saskatchewan that seeks to capture the Saskatchewan experience through an interactive archive, a repository of COVID news stories, and a timeline of the health policy decisions made throughout the pandemic.[34] The group has also launched an online memorial called "Remember Lives Not Numbers" that seeks to breathe life into the statistics by sharing the stories of those who have died from COVID in Saskatchewan.[35] Starting with the names and histories of people like Vic Thunderchild or Ali Syed whose deaths were known because of public reporting, the project offers people a place to share untold stories, keeping the memory of those they lost alive. Physical memorials, online and published histories, and books like this one are part of how we come to understand the depths of this experience and make it meaningful for those who follow.

Beyond these memories and reflections, people also deserve answers. Canada performed far better than some countries, far worse than others. Comparing ourselves with the United States is a national pastime, but that country tends to be an outlier, not a helpful norm by which to judge. The United States has the third-worst per capita COVID death rate in the world after Peru and Hungary. Canada is fifteenth, better than countries like France, the United Kingdom, and Sweden, but far worse than places like the Philippines, South Korea, Australia, and Japan.[36] We could have done worse, but we also could have done so much better. Canadians deserve a thorough and objective look back at what happened.

Asking the Hard Questions

And while we will want to examine our national response, one of the more striking realities of this crisis in Canada is that it was so clearly not a national response. When we hear of how other countries did – Vietnam, Peru, New Zealand, Sweden – you get the impression of a national standard, for better or worse. And perhaps within these countries they have the same sense of regional differences – that's difficult to say from abroad. What I can say is that the Canadian response calls into question the functionality of our federation when it comes to major challenges, leaving choices with national impact up to local governments. Each province was left to its own devices, with vastly different approaches and results. There is value in local autonomy and expertise in health, but in the face of a global crisis that model failed us. What kind of a country are we if we allow the people of one province to have such a vastly better or worse chance of making it through a health disaster than those of another region?

Federal health minister Jean-Yves Duclos's indication that a "broad review on Canada's pandemic response is coming"[37] is welcome news and will need to be complemented by or include reviews or inquiries at the provincial and territorial levels as well. Dr. David Naylor, who headed the 2003 SARS review that led to the establishment of the Public Health Agency of Canada,[38] has called for a national post-pandemic review led by international experts that includes an examination of federal and provincial gaps.[39] British Columbia completed a review, but it was limited to the operational response and largely excluded government and public health decisions.[40] In opposition, we first called for an inquiry into Saskatchewan's pandemic response in March 2021, asking for an nonpartisan, independent review of choices around testing and tracing, the response to the second wave, actions in long-term care, and the vaccine rollout.[41] After the disastrous events of the fourth wave we repeated that call,[42] but once again the government rejected the demand. *Regina Leader-Post* editor Russell Wangersky wrote at the time: "Sadly, a forward-looking government probably would have recognized the clear value of such a process and started a COVID inquiry on its own. But, because the provincial NDP suggested it, the inquiry baby is likely to be tossed out with the political bathwater."[43]

One can see why governments would be nervous about pulling back the curtain on what happened under their watch, but fear of political reprisal should not be a reason for people to accept a lack of transparency. Canadians appear to agree. Over 60 percent of respondents to an April 2022 cross-country opinion poll said they wanted to see a national inquiry and an inquiry in their own province.[44] This was independent of whether their province had performed poorly or well; people recognize that, as Wangersky wrote, "one of the ways to make sure that learning sticks – one of the ways to take advantage of all of that tragic COVID-19 education, with all of its heartbreak and loss – is to have a clear-eyed examination of what went right, and what went wrong."[45] And while some fingers will unavoidably be pointed, and some will find themselves taking responsibility for bad decisions, it shouldn't be about blame. What is more important is what we learn at a system level. Some have called for a pandemic amnesty, that we need to look to forgive and move forward.[46] That's a nice notion; I can get behind a pandemic amnesty, especially in our personal relations. But not pandemic amnesia. The purpose of telling our stories is not just to relive them, it's to use what we've learned from the past to change the future.

The COVID-19 pandemic has been a life-changing experience for us all, and one whose full effects we won't understand for a long time. This book presents some of the lessons we can and should learn. A recent article in *Nature*[47] identified similar themes around continued vigilance, vaccine-plus prevention, multi-sectoral collaboration, responsive health systems, combatting misinformation, and addressing health inequities. The lessons are becoming clearer, but the action needed to make change won't just happen. This experience demands that we make a conscious decision to not slip back into the past out of comfort or a desire to return to a normal that never was. There are things we can and must embrace about the way things were. There are others we must actively reject to leave space for a new approach. By examining what COVID-19 has revealed about what's wrong and what's right in our lives today, we can learn the lessons we need to build a healthy future.

Acknowledgments

This story and the lessons it teaches us have shifted as each wave of the pandemic has taken shape. I'm thankful to the team at UBC Press – and especially Nadine Pedersen, editor of the Purich Books imprint – for wise guidance and tremendous patience with each iteration.

As I wrote, I was welcomed into the lives of those who were willing to share their stories. I thank them for being willing to reopen their illness and grief in order that we all can learn from what they've been through. I have also drawn on the work of journalists, authors, and scientists who have performed the tremendous public service of chronicling and analyzing this rapidly changing and confusing period.

Irena Smith took on the daunting task of digging through the stories and research. This book would simply not have been possible without her insightful and diligent assistance. Dave Mitchell's wise advice and sharp edits made this a better project, as is always the case. Many friends and mentors have reviewed the book in whole or in part, and I thank them for their encouragement and support.

In my time in political life, I had the great fortune to work with candidates, MLAs, chiefs of staff, communications and research experts, party and caucus staff, constituency assistants, campaign managers, and countless volunteers. The list is too long, and the risk of leaving out someone I care deeply about too great, so I'll just say thank you. What incredible fortune it is to have the friendship of people who spend their time making the world a better place.

Mahli, Abe, and Gus pop up a lot in these pages, likely because I love them a lot and think about them all the time. I'm grateful to them for making life fun and meaningful, for permitting me to share our family's story, and for putting up with me through the pandemic, politics, and the writing of this book.

Notes

Foreword

1 Canadian Medical Association, "We Need to Mobilize Now: Alberta and Saskatchewan's Health Systems at Breaking Point," news release, September 29, 2021, https://www.cma.ca/news-releases-and-statements/we-need-mobilize-now-alberta-and-saskatchewans-health-systems-breaking.

2 Courtney Howard (@courtghoward), "[thank you emoji] to all who have encouraged me to run for the leadership of @CanadianGreens. I view political involvement as humanitarian work that is key to a #healthyfuture ...," Twitter, June 28, 2022, https://twitter.com/courtghoward/status/1541943238055104513.

Introduction

1 Zak Vescera, "COVID-19: Shahab Weeps While Presenting Modelling, Says Sask. at Turning Point," *Saskatoon StarPhoenix*, October 21, 2021, https://thestarphoenix.com/news/saskatchewan/covid-19-shahab-says-saskatchewan-at-fateful-turning-point.

2 Leyland Cecco, "Top Saskatchewan Official Moved to Tears by Unchecked Covid Spread," *Guardian*, October 21, 2021, https://www.theguardian.com/world/2021/oct/21/saskatchewan-health-official-tears-covid-vaccination.

3 Tedros Adhanom Ghebreyesus, "Achieving Health for All Requires Action on the Economic and Commercial Determinants of Health," *Lancet*, March 2023, https://doi.org/10.1016/s0140-6736(23)00574-3.

4 Rudolf Virchow, *Collected Essays on Public Health and Epidemiology* (Caton, MA: Science History Publications, 1985). Originally published 1879.

5 Ryan Meili, *A Healthy Society: How a Focus on Health Can Revive Canadian Democracy* (Saskatoon: Purich Publishing, 2012); Ryan Meili, *A Healthy Society: How a Focus on Health Can Revive Canadian Democracy, Updated and Expanded Edition* (Vancouver: Purich Books, 2018).

6 "Think Upstream," https://www.thinkupstream.ca.

7 "Division of Social Accountability," University of Saskatchewan College of Medicine, https://medicine.usask.ca/social-accountability/index.php.

8 Dennis Raphael, Toba Bryant, Juha Mikkonen, and Alexander Raphael, *Social Determinants of Health: The Canadian Facts*, 2nd ed. (Oshawa/Toronto: Ontario Tech University Faculty of Health Sciences/York University School of Health Policy and Management, 2020), http://thecanadianfacts.org.

9 Roy J. Romanow, "Accelerating the Third Revolution in Public Health Care" (speech given at Community Health Centres: Acting Today, Shaping Tomorrow conference, Toronto, June 10, 2011), https://uwaterloo.ca/canadian-index -wellbeing/sites/ca.canadian-index-wellbeing/files/uploads/files/2011-Third revolution_Romanow.pdf.

10 Tara J. Moriarty et al., *Excess All-Cause Mortality during the COVID-19 Epidemic in Canada* (Ottawa: Royal Society of Canada, 2021), https://rsc-src.ca/sites/ default/files/EM%20PB_EN.pdf.

FIRST WAVE

Total cases and deaths in Canada from Max Roser, Hannah Ritchie, Esteban Ortiz-Ospina, and Joe Hasell, "Coronavirus Pandemic (COVID-19)," *Our World in Data*, https://ourworldindata.org/coronavirus/country/canada. Total deaths in Saskatchewan from "Saskatchewan's Dashboard – Health and Wellness," Government of Saskatchewan, https://dashboard.saskatchewan. ca/health-wellness.

Gathering Clouds

1 "Coronavirus Could Move from Person to Person: WHO," *Saskatoon StarPhoenix*, January 15, 2020.

2 "Mystery Virus Causes Concern of Global Spread," *Saskatoon StarPhoenix*, January 10, 2020, NP4.

3 "The Epidemiology of HIV in Canada," CATIE, 2021, https://www.catie.ca/ the-epidemiology-of-hiv-in-canada.

4 Izn Shahab and Ryan Meili, "Examining Non-Attendance of Doctor's Appointments at a Community Clinic in Saskatoon," *Canadian Family Physician* 65, 6 (2019): e264–e268.

5 Legislative Assembly of Saskatchewan, *Debates and Proceedings*, 28th Leg., 4th Sess. (March 17, 2020) (Scott Moe, Saskatchewan Party), https://docs. legassembly.sk.ca/legdocs/Legislative%20Assembly/Hansard/28L4S/ 200317Debates.pdf.

6 Geoff Leo, "Saskatchewan Government Failed to Order Key Equipment and Supplies until after COVID-19 Arrived," *CBC News*, March 23, 2020, https:// www.cbc.ca/news/canada/saskatchewan/government-failed-to-order-key -covid-equipment-1.5506247.

7 Leo, "Saskatchewan Government Failed."

8   Brad Wall, "Foreword: Mandates and the Eight Most Powerful Words in Pol-
    itics," in *The Saskatchewan Election: A 2020 Perspective*, ed. Loleen Berdhal et al.
    (Regina/Saskatoon: Johnson Shoyama Graduate School of Public Policy, 2020).

9   Legislative Assembly of Saskatchewan, *Debates and Proceedings*, 26th Leg.,
    2nd Sess. (October 28, 2008) (Don Morgan, Saskatchewan Party), https://docs.
    legassembly.sk.ca/legdocs/Legislative%20Assembly/Hansard/26L2S/081028
    Hansard.pdf#page=29.

10 Arthur White-Crummey, "Election Booking Bumped Bid for COVID Testing
    Site in Regina School," *Regina Leader-Post*, July 3, 2020.

11 Carly Weeks, "Between 30 and 70 Percent of Canadians Could Become Infected
    with Coronavirus, Patty Hajdu Says," *Globe and Mail*, March 11, 2020, https://
    www.theglobeandmail.com/canada/article-between-30-and-70-per-cent-of
    -canadians-could-be-infected-with/.

12 *A Dictionary of Epidemiology*, ed. John M. Last, 4th ed. (Oxford: Oxford
    University Press, 2000), s.v. "pandemic."

13 James Shewaga, "USask Unites: VIDO-InterVac Team Tackles Coronavirus:
    Researchers Developing Prototype Vaccines at USask," *University of Sas-
    katchewan News*, March 13, 2020, https://news.usask.ca/articles/research/2020/
    vido-intervac-team-tackles-coronavirus-researchers-developing-prototype
    -vaccines-at-usask.php.

14 Stephanie Taylor, "Saskatchewan Premier Scott Moe Says Coronavirus Not a
    Factor in Election Call," *Global News*, March 3, 2020, https://globalnews.ca/
    news/6623374/scott-moe-coronavirus-saskatchewan-election-call/.

15 Legislative Assembly of Saskatchewan, *Debates and Proceedings*, 28th Leg.,
    4th Sess. (March 10, 2020) (Donna Harpauer, Saskatchewan Party), https://docs.
    legassembly.sk.ca/legdocs/Legislative%20Assembly/Hansard/28L4S/200310
    Debates.pdf.

16 Anne Huang (@drannehuang), "THREAD [downward pointing finger emoji]
    An open letter regarding the implications of an early #skpoli election on
    #COVID19 containment #cdnhealth @PremierScottMoe @ryanmeili
    ...," Twitter, March 9, 2020, https://twitter.com/drannehuang/status/
    1237079645264031744.

17 Laura Sciarpelletti, "Sask. Opposition Say Former Health Minister Lied about
    Province's COVID-19 Preparedness Plan in March 2020," *CBC News*, March
    11, 2021, https://www.cbc.ca/news/canada/saskatchewan/ndp-say-former
    -health-minister-lied-about-province-s-covid-19-preparedness-plan-in
    -march-2020-1.5946119.

18 J.P. Lewis and Robert Burroughs, "External Shocks and Westminster Gov-
    ernance: New Brunswick's All-Party Cabinet Committee on COVID-19,"
    Canadian Parliamentary Review 43, 3 (November 2020), http://www.revparlcan.
    ca/en/external-shocks-and-westminster-executive-governance-new
    -brunswicks-all-party-cabinet-committee-on-covid-19/.

19 Murray Mandryk, "Mandryk: Moe Should Bring Others into the Decision-
    Making Fold," *Regina Leader-Post*, March 24, 2020, https://leaderpost.com/

opinion/columnists/mandryk-moe-should-bring-others-into-the-decision-making-fold/wcm/57d0f1eb-a699-42e5-9b6d-74525966ce81/.

20 Howard Leeson, "Leeson: Governments Need to Re-organize Now to Face COVID-19 Crisis," *Saskatoon StarPhoenix*, April 3, 2020, https://thestarphoenix.com/opinion/columnists/leeson-governments-need-to-re-organize-now-to-face-covid-19-crisis/wcm/f41f2d3f-f0f2-4432-af87-f1ea670c2cfd/.

21 Murray Mandryk, "The Legislature Has Become a Better Place, a Quiet Place," *Regina Leader-Post*, March 17, 2020, https://leaderpost.com/opinion/columnists/mandryk-the-legislative-assembly-has-become-a-quiet-place-a-better-place.

The Longest March

1 Martin Turcotte, *Volunteering and Charitable Giving in Canada* (Ottawa: Statistics Canada, 2015), https://www150.statcan.gc.ca/n1/pub/89-652-x/89-652-x2015001-eng.htm#archived.

2 Theresa Tam (@CPHO_Canada), "2/2 @thelobbykb in Regina, SK, has teamed up with a local NGO to provide lunches to students who are food insecure and are missing regular meal programs ...," Twitter, March 26, 2020, https://twitter.com/CPHO_Canada/status/1243360925534408704.

3 Ian Gustafson, "Eleanor, the Golden Bread Winner," *PA Now*, April 8, 2020, https://panow.com/2020/04/08/eleanor-the-golden-bread-winner/.

4 Amanda Short, "Métis Nation – Saskatchewan Thanks Community Mask Makers with Supplies Donation," *Saskatoon StarPhoenix*, May 29, 2020, https://thestarphoenix.com/news/local-news/metis-nation-saskatchewan-thanks-community-mask-makers-with-supplies-donation.

5 Catherine Porter, "The Top Doctor Who Aced the Coronavirus Test," *New York Times*, June 5, 2020, https://www.nytimes.com/2020/06/05/world/canada/bonnie-henry-british-columbia-coronavirus.html; Amy Judd and Richard Zussman, "Dr. Henry Shoes Sell Out as Fluevog Website Crashes Amidst Excitement," *Global News*, April 23, 2020, https://globalnews.ca/news/6860502/bonnie-henry-shoe-john-fluevog-presale-start-thursday/.

6 Arthur White-Crummey, "Dr. Saqib Shahab Relishes the 'Simple Pleasures' of Family as He Outworks the Virus," *Regina Leader-Post*, June 5, 2020.

7 White-Crummey, "Dr. Saqib Shahab."

8 "Ryan Meili's #stayhome staylist," Spotify, https://open.spotify.com/playlist/0FAy5roaLLQFdmBUXw5kD4?si=wsIYuTWQR3uzCJaDz2KYPg&nd=1.

9 Guy Quenneville, Stefani Langenegger, and Adam Hunter, "COVID-19 in Sask: Internal Draft Gov't Document Outlines 'Worst Case Scenario' of up to 15,000 Deaths," *CBC News*, March 24, 2020, https://www.cbc.ca/news/canada/saskatoon/saskatchewan-coronavirus-1.5507892; Saskatchewan Health Authority, "COVID-19 Planning: Strategy for Continuity of Health Services and Surge Capacity" (PowerPoint presentation, March 19, 2020), https://www.documentcloud.org/documents/6818248-SHA-COVID-19-Service-Continuity-and-Surge-Plan.html.

10 J. Kottke, "The Paradox of Preparation," Kottke.org, March 16, 2020, https://kottke.org/20/03/the-paradox-of-preparation.

11 Andrew Green, "A Tribute to Some of the Doctors Who Died from COVID-19," *Lancet* 396, 10264 (November 2020): 1720–29, https://doi.org/10.1016/S0140-6736(20)32478-8.

Losing Trust

1 Canadian Press, "Saskatchewan Premier Says He Wouldn't Change a Thing about COVID-19 Response," *CBC News*, December 30, 2020, https://www.cbc.ca/news/canada/saskatchewan/sask-premier-says-he-wouldnt-change-covid-19-response-1.5857238.

2 David Holt, "In Praise of Those Who Resist Temptation," *Bulwark*, January 4, 2021, https://www.thebulwark.com/in-praise-of-those-who-resist-temptation/.

3 COVID-19 National Preparedness Collaborators, "Pandemic Preparedness and COVID-19: An Exploratory Analysis of Infection and Fatality Rates, and Contextual Factors Associated with Preparedness in 177 Countries, from Jan 1, 2020, to Sept 30, 2021," *Lancet* 399, 10334 (April 2022): 1489–512, https://doi.org/10.1016/S0140-6736(22)00172-6.

4 Evan Dyer, "Some Health Experts Questioning Advice against Wider Use of Masks to Slow Spread of COVID-19," *CBC News*, March 31, 2020, https://www.cbc.ca/news/politics/covid-19-pandemic-coronavirus-masks-1.5515526.

5 "Story," #Masks4All, https://masks4all.org/story.

6 Ryan Meili, "Masks and COVID-19," video, 4:01, April 5, 2020, https://www.youtube.com/watch?v=bgtYcwod6jo.

7 John Paul Tasker, "Canada's Top Doctor Says Non-Medical Masks Can Help Stop the Spread of COVID-19," *CBC News*, April 6, 2020, https://www.cbc.ca/news/politics/non-medical-masks-covid-19-spread-1.5523321.

8 Ryan Meili (@ryanmeili), "Saskatchewan people are asking politicians to put aside their differences and work together right now. This is the letter I wrote to @PremierSottMoe today," Twitter, April 7, 2020, 4:14 p.m., https://twitter.com/ryanmeili/status/1247663959802609665.

9 "Advocacy," Saskatoon Inter-Agency Response to COVID-19, https://saskatooninteragencyresponse.ca/advocacy/.

10 Bryan Eneas, "Clawing Back of CERB Payments Will Hurt Poorest in Sask.: Anti-Poverty Advocate," *CBC News*, September 24, 2020, https://www.cbc.ca/news/canada/saskatchewan/clawing-back-cerb-hurt-poorest-1.5737345.

11 Tracey Tong, "Dr. Naheed Dosani Started PEACH to Provide Palliative Care for Homeless and Vulnerable Housed Populations," *Toronto Star*, August 8, 2021, https://www.thestar.com/life/together/people/2021/08/08/dr-naheed-dosani-started-peach-to-provide-palliative-care-for-homeless-and-vulnerably-housed-populations.html.

12 Naheed Dosani, "Nurturing Better Health Outcomes through Equity," *Ontario Medical Review*, April 2021, https://www.oma.org/newsroom/ontario-medical

-review/archived-issues/spring-2021/nurturing-better-health-outcomes-through
-equity/.

13 Alexandra Mae Jones, "Shelter Outbreaks Leave People Experiencing Home-lessness Even More Vulnerable during COVID-19," *CTV News*, March 21, 2021, https://www.ctvnews.ca/canada/shelter-outbreaks-leave-people-experiencing
-homelessness-even-more-vulnerable-during-covid-19-1.5356600.

14 Amanda Short, "COVID-19 Outbreak Declared at the Lighthouse, First at a Shelter in the Province," *Saskatoon StarPhoenix*, October 25, 2020.

Reopening Minds

1   Stephanie Taylor, "'We Have Flattened the Curve:' Saskatchewan May Reopen Some Businesses in May," *Toronto Star*, April 22, 2020, https://www.thestar.com/news/canada/2020/04/22/we-have-flattened-the-curve-saskatchewan-may
-reopen-some-businesses-in-may.html.

2   Guy Quenneville and Adam Hunter, "COVID-19 in Sask: Top Doc 'Extremely Happy' with Low Case Numbers but Says Province Needs to Avoid 2nd wave," *CBC News*, April 14, 2020, https://www.cbc.ca/news/canada/saskatoon/coronavirus-saskatchewan-1.5531567.

3   Tomas Pueyo, "Coronavirus: The Hammer and the Dance," *Medium*, March 19, 2020, https://tomaspueyo.medium.com/coronavirus-the-hammer-and
-the-dance-be9337092b56.

4   Pueyo, "Coronavirus."

5   Hannah Ritchie et al., "Coronavirus (COVID-19) Deaths," *Our World in Data*, https://ourworldindata.org/covid-deaths#citation.

6   Kanoko Matsuyama and James Mayger, "How Japan Achieved One of the World's Lowest Covid-19 Death Rates," *Business Standard*, June 18, 2022, https://www.business-standard.com/article/international/how-is-japan-s-covid-death
-rate-lowest-among-wealthiest-nations-in-world-122061800170_1.html.

7   Sophie Cousins, "New Zealand Eliminates COVID-19," *Lancet* 395, 10235 (May 7, 2020): 1474.

8   Ryan Meili, "Meili: Reopening Plan Has to Put People First," *Saskatoon StarPhoenix*, April 23, 2020, https://thestarphoenix.com/opinion/columnists/meili-reopening-plan-has-to-put-people-first/wcm/56ce7354-f88a-466b-8beb
-713a8e2115d9/.

9   Bonnie Allen, "Largest Outbreak of COVID-19 in an Indigenous Community in Canada Offers Important Lessons," *CBC News*, September 29, 2020, https://www.cbc.ca/news/canada/saskatchewan/outbreak-covid-19-indigenous
-community-lessons-1.5737126.

10 "Home," The 155 Collective, https://www.the155.ca/.

11 Derek Ruttle, "Outlook Native Turned Doctor Recognized for Leadership," *SaskToday.ca*, November 18, 2021, https://www.sasktoday.ca/central/outlook/outlook-native-turned-doctor-recognized-for-leadership-4773862.

12 Jason Warick, "Inaccurate, Unfair for Sask. Premier to Single Out Northern First Nations on Vaccination, Say Critics," *CBC News*, September 24, 2021,

https://www.cbc.ca/news/canada/saskatoon/northern-first-nations-covid-19
-scott-moe-1.6187634.

13 Jetet Heer, "Reckoning with a Year of Shared Isolation, Pandemic, and Protest," *Nation*, February 26, 2021, https://www.thenation.com/article/society/covid
-anniversary-gramsci-sorel/.

14 Mickey Djuric, "Anti-Mask Rallies Held in Saskatchewan as COVID-19 Cases Rise," *Global News*, July 19, 2020, https://globalnews.ca/news/7195233/
coronavirus-saskatoon-regina-anti-mask-rallies/.

15 Jack Hicks, "Opinion: Sask. Suicide Prevention Strategy a 'Travesty,'" *Regina Leader-Post*, May 20, 2020, https://leaderpost.com/opinion/columnists/opinion
-sask-suicide-prevention-strategy-a-travesty/wcm/e3041b85-ce2d-4118-a81c
-fb83d7e5b247/.

16 Allison Crawford, "A National Suicide Prevention Strategy for Canadians – From Research to Policy and Practice," *Canadian Journal of Psychiatry* 60, 6 (June 2015): 239–41; Federation of Sovereign Indigenous Nations, *Saskatchewan First Nations Suicide Prevention Strategy* (Saskatoon: Federation of Sovereign Indigenous Nation, 2018), https://www.suicideinfo.ca/wp-content/uploads/
gravity_forms/6-191a85f36ce9e20de2e2fa3869197735/2018/07/Saskatchewan
-First-Nations-Suicide-Prevention-Strategy_oa.pdf.

17 Jack Hicks, "Saints or Sinners on Suicide Prevention?" *Regina Leader-Post*, May 5, 2019, https://leaderpost.com/opinion/columnists/saints-or-sinners-on
-suicide-prevention.

18 "Pillars for Life: Saskatchewan's Suicide Prevention Plan," Government of Saskatchewan, https://www.saskatchewan.ca/government/health-care
-administration-and-provider-resources/saskatchewan-health-initiatives/
suicide-prevention-plan.

19 Zak Vescera, "Expert, MLA Say Sask. Suicide Prevention Plan Misses the Mark," *Saskatoon StarPhoenix*, May 13, 2020, https://thestarphoenix.com/news/local
-news/mla-who-pushed-for-suicide-prevention-bill-says-gov-plan-not-enough/
wcm/04b0e924-4f87-48c7-b17b-cc602b6efda3/.

20 Chelsea Laskowski, "'We Are Hurting': As Sask. First Nations Grapple with Suicides, Feds Announce \$2.5M in Prevention Funding," *CBC News*, December 19, 2019, https://www.cbc.ca/news/canada/saskatoon/suicide-prevention
-crisis-ochapowace-1.5403081.

21 "'It's Difficult to Understand': Hospital Staff Testify at Samwel Uko Inquest," *CBC News*, June 2, 2022, https://www.cbc.ca/news/canada/saskatchewan/
samwel-uko-inquest-enters-fourth-day-1.6475521.

22 Ashley Martin, "NDP Calls for Public Inquiry into Saskatchewan's High Rates of Suicide," *Regina Leader-Post*, August 10, 2020, https://leaderpost.com/news/
local-news/ndp-calls-for-public-inquiry-into-saskatchewans-high-rates-of
-suicide.

23 Guy Quenneville, "Tristen Durocher Vows to Remain in Wascana Park until Planned End of Ceremonial Fast on Sept. 13," *CBC News*, August 11, 2020, https://www.cbc.ca/news/canada/saskatoon/suicide-awareness-hunger
-strike-tristen-durocher-1.5681532.

24   Jennifer Francis, "Tristen Durocher Ends 44-Day Fast, Takes Down Teepee Camp at Wascana Park," *CBC News*, September 13, 2020, https://www.cbc.ca/news/canada/saskatchewan/durocher-ends-44-day-fast-takes-down-teepee-1.5722669.

25   Zak Vescera, "Creator of Sask. Suicide Prevention Law Says Government Is Failing to Follow It," *Saskatoon StarPhoenix*, April 27, 2022, https://thestarphoenix.com/news/saskatchewan/creator-of-sask-suicide-prevention-law-says-government-is-failing-to-follow-it.

26   Daniella Ponticelli, "Sask. Govt Rejects Call from Families, Opposition for Mental Health Committee," *CBC News*, May 18, 2022, https://www.cbc.ca/news/canada/saskatchewan/suicide-prevention-special-committee-1.6457300.

27   Michael Bramadat-Willcock, "'Let It Burn': Activist Likens Suicide Prevention Policy to Ignoring Forest Fires," *SaskToday.ca*, August 13, 2020, https://www.sasktoday.ca/north/local-news/let-it-burn-activist-likens-suicide-prevention-policy-to-ignoring-forest-fires-4153810.

28   Paul Smetanin et al., *The Life and Economic Impact of Major Mental Illnesses in Canada* (Toronto: RiskAnalytica, on behalf of the Mental Health Commission of Canada, 2011), https://www.mentalhealthcommission.ca/wp-content/uploads/drupal/MHCC_Report_Base_Case_FINAL_ENG_0_0.pdf.

29   Smetanin et al., *Life and Economic Impact*.

30   World Health Organization, "Mental Health and COVID-19: Early Evidence of the Pandemic's Impact," March 2, 2022, https://apps.who.int/iris/bitstream/handle/10665/352189/WHO-2019-nCoV-Sci-Brief-Mental-health-2022.1-eng.pdf.

Eye of the Storm

1   Arthur White-Crummey, "Meili and Notley Rev Up NDP Troops as Campaign Enters Home Stretch," *Regina Leader-Post*, October 23, 2020, https://leaderpost.com/news/politics/sask-election/meili-and-notley-rev-up-ndp-troops-as-campaign-enters-home-stretch.

2   Scott Moe (@PremierScottMoe), "Even though Justin Trudeau recently said Canada is now in the second wave of COVID-19, I remain confident we can avoid a significant second wave here ...," Twitter, September 26, 2020, https://twitter.com/premierscottmoe/status/1309871011249053696.

3   Saskatchewan's NDP Caucus, *A People-First Recovery* (Regina: Saskatchewan NDP, 2020), https://d3n8a8pro7vhmx.cloudfront.net/saskndp/mailings/3164/attachments/original/A_People-First_Recovery_-_Sask_NDP.pdf?1591902056.

4   Stephanie Taylor, "Saskatchewan Headed for Austerity as It Deals with $2.1B COVID-19 Deficit," *Toronto Star*, August 27, 2020, https://www.thestar.com/business/2020/08/27/saskatchewan-to-provide-first-covid-19-deficit-update-future-outlook.html.

5   New Democrats, *People First: Platform 2020* (September 2020), https://www.saskndp.ca/platform_pdf.

6   "Closing the Gap," Government of Australia, https://www.closingthegap.gov.au/.

7   "Moms Stop the Harm Board of Directors," https://www.momsstoptheharm. com/team.

8   Lynn Giesbrecht, "Moe Makes Final Regina Campaign Stop, Promises No Second Lockdown," *Regina Leader-Post,* October 24, 2020, https://leaderpost. com/news/politics/sask-election/moe-makes-final-regina-campaign-stop -promises-no-second-lockdown.

9   Brian Zinchuk, "Moe Discusses New Mandate, but Is Questioned on Buffalo Party Performance," *Toronto Star,* October 28, 2020, https://www.thestar.com/ news/canada/2020/10/28/moe-discusses-new-mandate-but-is-questioned-on -buffalo-party-performance.html.

SECOND WAVE

Total cases and deaths in Canada from Max Roser, Hannah Ritchie, Esteban Ortiz-Ospina, and Joe Hasell, "Coronavirus Pandemic (COVID-19)," *Our World in Data,* https://ourworldindata.org/coronavirus/country/canada. Total deaths in Saskatchewan from "Saskatchewan's Dashboard – Health and Wellness," Government of Saskatchewan, https://dashboard.saskatchewan. ca/health-wellness.

Ignoring the Signs

1   Mike Ives, "Fred Sasakamoose, One of the First Indigenous N.H.L. Players, Dies at 86," *New York Times,* December 5, 2020, https://www.nytimes. com/2020/12/05/obituaries/fred-sasakamoose-dead-coronavirus.html/.

2   Fred Sasakamoose, *Call Me Indian: From the Trauma of Residential School to Becoming the NHL's First Treaty Indigenous Player* (Toronto: Penguin Canada, 2021).

3   Zak Vescera, "First Nations Launch Vaccination Clinics for Urban Members," *Saskatoon StarPhoenix,* April 5, 2021, https://thestarphoenix.com/news/ saskatchewan/first-nations-launch-vaccination-clinics-for-urban-members.

4   Arthur White-Crummey, "Post-Election Modelling Showed Early Risk of Huge COVID Wave in Sask.," *Regina Leader-Post,* January 9, 2021, https:// leaderpost.com/news/saskatchewan/post-election-modelling-showed-early -risk-of-huge-covid-wave-in-sask.

5   Arthur White-Crummey, "New Modelling Shows Stark Risk of COVID Inaction in Sask.," *Regina Leader-Post,* November 18, 2020, https://leaderpost. com/news/saskatchewan/new-modelling-shows-stark-risk-of-covid-inaction -in-sask.

6   Peter Lozinski, "Updated COVID-19 Modelling Data Shows Impact of Public Health Measures," *Prince Albert Daily Herald,* November 19, 2020, https:// paherald.sk.ca/updated-covid-19-modelling-data-shows-impact-of-public -health-measures/.

7   Saskatchewan NDP Caucus, "NDP Calls for 'Circuit Breaker' of Non-Essential Services to Protect Businesses and Healthcare System," news release, November 18, 2020, https://www.ndpcaucus.sk.ca/circuit_breaker.

8 Jason Warick, "'We Are Losing This Battle': More Than 300 Sask. Doctors Sign Letter Demanding Government Action on COVID-19," *CBC News*, November 11, 2020, https://www.cbc.ca/news/canada/saskatoon/doctors-open-letter-1.5797316.

9 Brent Thoma (@Brent_Thoma), "@PremierScottMoe Our positivity rate is at 8.2%. Case numbers are exploding. We are losing. With respect, 346 Saskatchewan physicians are asking you to step up ...," Twitter, November 11, 2020, https://twitter.com/brent_thoma/status/1326625814381694976.

10 Nicholas Frew, "Masks Mandatory in More Indoor Public Spaces in Sask., Curfew on Alcohol Sales Coming Monday," *CBC News*, November 13, 2020, https://www.cbc.ca/news/canada/saskatchewan/saskatchewan-covid-19-update-1.5800809.

11 Brent Thoma (@Brent_Thoma), "In follow-up to our first letter, many asked what physicians think SK should do. We hoped that the announcement today would make this redundant ... It didn't ...," Twitter, November 13, 2020, https://twitter.com/Brent_Thoma/status/1327332794666606592?ref_src=twsrc%5Etfw.

12 Saskatchewan Medical Association, "Health Organizations Unite in Call for Additional COVID-19 Measures," news release, November 13, 2020, https://www.srna.org/wp-content/uploads/2020/11/SRNA-SMA-Call-for-Additional-COVID-Measures.pdf.

13 Heidi Atter, "197 Sask. Doctors Sign Open Letter Asking Businesses to Do More to Stop Coronavirus Spread," *CBC News*, March 19, 2020, https://www.cbc.ca/news/canada/saskatchewan/sask-doctor-letter-businesses-coronavirus-1.5502582.

14 Arthur White-Crummey, "Changemakers: Hassan Masri Fights COVID-19 and Misinformation in Sask.," *Regina Leader-Post*, March 15, 2021, https://leaderpost.com/news/postpandemic/changemakers-hassan-masri-fights-covid-19-and-misinformation-in-sask.

15 Yasmine Ghania, "Sask. ICU Doctor Leaving Province Partly Due to Premier Moe's 'Failed Leadership' during Pandemic," *CBC News*, May 13, 2022, https://www.cbc.ca/news/canada/saskatchewan/sask-icu-doctor-leaving-province-partly-over-premier-moe-s-failed-leadership-during-pandemic-1.6452760.

16 "Health Advocate," Royal College of Physicians and Surgeons of Canada, https://www.royalcollege.ca/rcsite/canmeds/framework/canmeds-role-health-advocate-e.

17 "Advocacy Group Starts COVID-19 Briefings to 'Fill the Void' Left by Alberta Government Officials," *CBC News*, August 30, 2021, https://www.cbc.ca/news/canada/calgary/vipond-protect-our-province-covid-1.6158546.

18 Miranda Caley, "Burlington Doctor Uses Her Online Voice to Ease Public's Fears and Influence Policy," *Healthy Debate*, October 15, 2021, https://healthydebate.ca/2021/10/topic/burlington-doctor-uses-her-online-voice-to-ease-publics-fears-and-influence-policy/; "Ontario's Long-Term Care Sector Is in a Grave Humanitarian Crisis," Doctors for Justice in LTC, https://docs4ltcjustice.ca/.

19 "'Slap in the Face': Sask. Premier's Advice to Medical Workers Hits Sour Note with Doctor," *CTV News*, September 22, 2021, https://saskatoon.ctvnews.ca/

slap-in-the-face-sask-premier-s-advice-to-medical-workers-hits-sour-note-with
-doctor-1.5596172.

20 Patrick Fafard, Brittany McNena, Agatha Suszek, and Steven J. Hoffman,
    "Contested Roles of Canada's Chief Medical Officers of Health," *Canadian
    Journal of Public Health* 109 (2018): 587–88, https://doi.org/10.17269/
    s41997-018-0080-3.

21 Sarath Peiris, "Opinion: Medical Health Officers Should Be Fully Independent,"
    Saskatoon StarPhoenix, August 24, 2021, https://thestarphoenix.com/opinion/
    columnists/opinion-medical-health-officers-should-be-fully-independent.

22 Brian Zinchuk, "Moe, Meili, Condemn Speaker at Regina 'Freedom Rally'
    for Disparaging Dr. Shahab," *SaskToday.ca*, December 14, 2020, https://www.
    sasktoday.ca/north/local-news/moe-meili-condemn-speaker-at-regina
    -freedom-rally-for-disparaging-dr-shahab-4160412.

23 "Premier Condemns Protest Outside Saskatchewan Chief Medical Officer's
    Home," *CBC News*, January 24, 2021, https://www.cbc.ca/news/canada/
    saskatchewan/premier-moe-condems-protest-shahab-1.5885638.

24 Adeoluwa Atayero, "Sask. Opposition Calls on Province to Take Action against
    Hospital Protests," *CBC News*, September 15, 2020, https://www.cbc.ca/news/
    canada/saskatchewan/oppositions-moe-action-record-breaking-hospitalizations
    -1.6176745; Yasmine Ghania and Adam Hunter, "Saskatchewan Introduces Legis-
    lation Banning COVID Protesters around Hospitals," *CBC News*, November
    10, 2021, https://www.cbc.ca/news/canada/saskatchewan/hospital-covid-protest
    -buffer-zone-1.6244087.

25 Laura Sciarpelletti, "Regina Tim Hortons Team Makes Tribute to Top Doctor
    with Sweater Vest Donut," *CBC News*, February 3, 2021, https://www.cbc.ca/
    news/canada/saskatchewan/regina-tim-hortons-team-tribute-doctor-sweater
    -vest-donut-1.5899532.

26 Peiris, "Opinion: Medical Health Officers."

27 Murray Mandryk, "Dr. Shahab Should Report Directly to Sask. Legislature,"
    Regina Leader-Post, April 9, 2023, https://leaderpost.com/opinion/columnists/
    murray-mandryk-dr-shahab-should-report-directly-to-sask-legislature.

Back to School

1   Vic Thunderchild (@vic65tc), Twitter, April 5, 2021, https://twitter.com/
    VicThunderchild/status/1379163208028618752.

2   Mickey Djuric, "Saskatchewan Leaves Teachers, Other Front-Line Workers
    Off Its Vaccine Priority List," *CBC News*, April 14, 2021, https://www.cbc.ca/
    news/canada/saskatchewan/saskatchewan-leaves-teachers-other-front-line
    -workers-off-its-vaccine-priority-list-1.5987564.

3   Michael Lewis, *The Premonition* (New York: W.W. Norton, 2021), 87.

4   Nicole Racine, Brae Anne McArthur, and Jessica E. Cooke, "Global Prevalence
    of Depressive and Anxiety Symptoms in Children and Adolescents during
    COVID-19: A Meta-Analysis," *JAMA Pediatrics* 175, 11 (2021): 1142–50, doi:10.1001/
    jamapediatrics.2021.2482.

5 Researchers under the Scope, "The Kids Are Not All Right, with Ayisha Kurji," University of Saskatchewan College of Medicine, January 17, 2022, https://medicine.usask.ca/news/2022/the-kids-are-not-all-right,-with-ayisha-kurji.php.

6 Wesley J. Park and Kristen A. Walsh, "COVID-19 and the Unseen Pandemic of Child Abuse," *BMJ Paediatrics Open* 6, 1 (2022): e001553, http://dx.doi.org/10.1136/bmjpo-2022-001553.

7 Robert Sege and Allison Stephens, "Child Physical Abuse Did Not Increase during the Pandemic," *JAMA Pediatrics* 176, 4 (2022): 338–40, doi:10.1001/jamapediatrics.2021.5476.

8 Sege and Stephens, "Child Physical Abuse."

9 H. Juliette T. Unwin et al., "Global, Regional, and National Minimum Estimates of Children Affected by COVID-19-Associated Orphanhood and Caregiver Death, by Age and Family Circumstance up to Oct 31, 2021: An Updated Modelling Study," *Lancet Child and Adolescent Health* (February 2022), https://doi.org/10.1016/s2352-4642(22)00005-0.

10 Clint Smith, "800,000 Deaths," *The Atlantic,* December 14, 2021, https://www.theatlantic.com/ideas/archive/2021/12/america-800000-dead-covid-19/620997/.

11 Zak Vescera, "Saskatchewan's ICUs Face Down Another COVID-19 Wave," *Saskatoon StarPhoenix,* April 9, 2021, https://thestarphoenix.com/news/saskatchewan/saskatchewans-icus-face-down-another-covid-19-wave.

12 Ruth Grimes to Scott Moe, Paul Merriman, and Saqib Shahab, on behalf of the Canadian Pediatric Society, October 4, 2022, https://cps.ca/uploads/advocacy/Protecting_children_and_youth_during_the_COVID_crisis_in_SK.Public_.pdf.

13 Mickey Djuric, "Saskatchewan Monitoring COVID-19 Measures Needed to Keep Essential Workers Healthy," *Toronto Star,* January 5, 2022, https://www.thestar.com/news/canada/2022/01/05/saskatchewan-monitoring-covid-19-measures-needed-to-keep-essential-workers-healthy.html.

14 Miguel Sanchez, *Saskatchewan Child and Family Poverty Report 2021* (Regina: University of Regina, 2021), https://campaign2000.ca/wp-content/uploads/2021/11/Saskatchewan-Report-Card-English-CPR-2021.pdf.

15 Courtney Carlberg and Jen Budney, *Saskatchewan's Failing Report Card on Child Care* (Regina: Canadian Centre for Policy Alternatives, 2019), https://policyalternatives.ca/publications/reports/saskatchewans-failing-report-card-child-care.

16 Saskatoon Public Schools, "Budget 2021–22," infographic, https://www.spsd.sk.ca/Documents/SPS%20Budget%20Infographic.pdf.

17 Alex MacPherson, "Top Stories of 2020: Teachers' Strike Avoided as Pandemic Surged into Saskatchewan," *Saskatoon StarPhoenix,* December 18, 2020, https://thestarphoenix.com/news/local-news/top-stories-of-2020-teachers-strike-avoided-as-pandemic-surged-into-saskatchewan.

18 Saskatchewan NDP Caucus, "Saskatchewan NDP Sets Out Back-to-School Priorities as COVID-19 Cases Rise," news release, July 29, 2020, https://www.ndpcaucus.sk.ca/saskatchewan_ndp_sets_out_back_to_school_priorities.

19 Theresa Kliem and Alicia Bridges, "Ventilation Guidelines Not Included in Sask. Back-to-School Plan," *CBC News*, August 13, 2020, https://www.cbc.ca/news/canada/saskatchewan/ventilation-guidelines-not-included-in-back-to-school-plan-1.5684431.

20 Lynn Giesbrecht, "Sask. Hits Record Number of Kids in Hospital with COVID-19," *Regina Leader-Post*, October 23, 2021, https://leaderpost.com/news/saskatchewan/sask-hits-record-high-number-of-kids-in-hospital-with-covid-19.

21 Caroline Alphonso, "Regina Public Schools Move from In-Class to Online, Raising Concerns of Learning Loss," *Globe and Mail*, December 13, 2020, https://www.theglobeandmail.com/canada/article-regina-schools-begin-remote-learning/; Lynn Giesbrecht, "Staff Shortages Have Regina Public Scrambling, High Schools Go Online Temporarily," *Regina Leader-Post*, January 18, 2022, https://leaderpost.com/news/local-news/regina-public-moves-all-high-schools-online-for-several-days.

22 Grimes to Moe, Merriman, and Shahab.

23 Grimes to Moe, Merriman, and Shahab.

24 Giesbrecht, "Sask. Hits Record Number."

25 André Picard, "Kids Are Suffering from COVID in Ways We Never Expected," *Globe and Mail*, November 7, 2022, https://www.theglobeandmail.com/opinion/article-kids-are-suffering-from-covid-in-ways-we-never-expected/; Janice Hopkins Tanne, "US Faces Triple Epidemic of Flu, RSV, and Covid," *BMJ* 379 (2022), https://doi.org/10.1136/bmj.o2681.

26 Elizabeth Payne, "CHEO Chief of Staff Pleads for Residents to Wear Masks to Protect Children as It Deals with Surge in Care Needs," *Ottawa Citizen*, November 8, 2022, https://ottawacitizen.com/news/local-news/cheo-chief-of-staff-pleads-for-residents-to-wear-masks-to-protect-children-as-it-deals-with-surge-in-care-needs.

27 Julia Wong, "Fewer than 7% of Kids 5 and Younger Have Gotten a COVID-19 Vaccine," *CBC News*, November 8, 2022, https://www.cbc.ca/news/canada/edmonton/covid19-vaccination-kids-under-five-low-1.6641727.

28 "Saskatoon Public Schools to Charge Fees for Lunch-Hour Supervision, Cut Teaching Jobs to Balance Books," *CBC News*, June 8, 2022, https://www.cbc.ca/news/canada/saskatoon/public-schools-supervision-charge-teachers-cut-balance-books-1.6481484.

29 Meghan Grant, "'Unreasonable' Order Lifting Alberta School Mask Mandate Made by Politicians Not Hinshaw: Judge," *CBC News*, October 27, 2022, https://www.cbc.ca/news/canada/calgary/school-mask-mandate-alberta-unreasonable-judge-decision-lagrange-1.6631695.

30 Jessie Anton, "Sask. Government Tightens Grip on School Divisions, Legally Directs All to Drop Mandates," *CBC News*, February 15, 2022, https://www.cbc.ca/news/canada/saskatchewan/sask-minister-letter-schools-drop-covid-mandates-1.6351865.

31 Alheli Picazo (@a_picazo), "Ontario: 'You can't mandate masking forever. Do your own risk assessment ...,'" Twitter, March 11, 2022, https://twitter.com/a_picazo/status/1502352454515662851.

32 Juliette Baxter, "The Outlook for Teachers Remains Challenging," *Globe and Mail*, October 22, 2022, https://www.theglobeandmail.com/life/article-the-outlook-for-teachers-remains-challenging/.

33 Sean Amato, "'Disrespected and Demoralized': Survey Shows 37% of Alberta Teachers May Leave in the Next Five Years," *CTV News*, January 27, 2022, https://edmonton.ctvnews.ca/disrespected-and-demoralized-survey-shows-37-of-alberta-teachers-may-leave-in-the-next-five-years-1.5757753.

34 Jason G. Antonio, "Forty-One Per Cent of Teachers Have Thought of Quitting Due to Burnout, NDP Survey Shows," *Moose Jaw Today*, October 21, 2019, https://www.moosejawtoday.com/local-news/forty-one-per-cent-of-teachers-have-thought-of-quitting-due-to-burnout-ndp-survey-shows-1756617.

35 Joe Vipond and Amanda Hu, "Opinion: Better Protecting Schools from COVID Is Within Reach," *Edmonton Journal*, August 17, 2022, https://edmontonjournal.com/opinion/columnists/opinion-better-protecting-schools-from-covid-is-within-reach/wcm/7ac5c39b-c958-4b44-9d03-a0e1b259ac0d/amp/.

Respecting Our Elders

1 Canadian Institute for Health Information, *Pandemic Experience in the Long-Term Care Sector: How Does Canada Compare with Other Countries?* (Ottawa: CIHI, 2020), https://www.cihi.ca/sites/default/files/document/covid-19-rapid-response-long-term-care-snapshot-en.pdf.

2 C.J.J. Mialowski to Sylvia Jones, May 14, 2020, https://www.macleans.ca/wp-content/uploads/2020/05/JTFC-Observations-in-LTCF-in-ON.pdf.

3 André Picard, *Neglected No More: The Urgent Need to Improve the Lives of Canada's Elders in the Wake of a Pandemic* (Toronto: Random House, 2021), 2.

4 Ariana Eunjung Cha and Dan Keating, "Covid Becomes Plague of Elderly, Reviving Debate over 'Acceptable Loss,'" *Washington Post*, November 28, 2022, https://www.washingtonpost.com/health/2022/11/28/covid-who-is-dying/.

5 Stephanie Thomas, "Concern Arises over Premier's 'Influenza' Comments, Focus on Seniors Death," *CTV News*, May 29, 2020, https://calgary.ctvnews.ca/concern-arises-over-premier-s-influenza-comments-focus-on-seniors-death-1.4959251.

6 Bobbi-Jean MacKinnon, "N.B.'s COVID-19 Deaths under 80 Higher Than National Average, Says Researcher," *CBC News*, June 17, 2022, https://www.cbc.ca/news/canada/new-brunswick/covid-19-deaths-new-brunswick-under-80-tara-moriarty-1.6492275.

7 Tracy Kidder, *Mountains beyond Mountains: The Quest of Dr. Paul Farmer, a Man Who Would Cure the World* (New York: Random House, 2003), 294.

8 Rachel Aiello, "'We Failed the Most Vulnerable': Dr. Tam's Biggest Takeaway after a Year of COVID-19," *CTV News*, March 14, 2021, https://www.ctvnews.ca/health/coronavirus/we-failed-the-most-vulnerable-dr-tam-s-biggest-takeaway-after-a-year-of-covid-19-1.5345393.

9 Aiello, "'We Failed the Most Vulnerable.'"

10 Kathleen Harris and Ashley Burke, "The Long-Term Care Crisis: How B.C. Controlled COVID-19 while Ontario, Quebec Face Disaster," *CBC News*, May

28, 2020, https://www.cbc.ca/news/politics/long-term-care-crisis-covid19
-pandemic-1.5589097.

11 Arthur White-Crummey and Lynn Giesbrecht, "Take Care; Pandemic Is Sask's
Best Chance for Change in Long-Term Care," *Regina Leader-Post,* March 6,
2021, https://leaderpost.com/news/saskatchewan/take-care-pandemic-is
-sask-s-best-chance-for-change-in-long-term-care.

12 "Malnourished Senior Concerns Raised at Legislature," *CBC News,* November
18, 2014, https://www.cbc.ca/news/canada/saskatchewan/malnourished-senior
-concerns-raised-at-legislature-1.2841012.

13 Jonathan Ore, "As Pressures Mount on Home Care in Canada, Experts Look
Abroad for Solutions," *CBC Radio,* September 17, 2022, https://www.cbc.ca/
radio/whitecoat/home-care-problems-solutions-wcba-1.6581490.

14 Legislative Assembly of Saskatchewan, *Debates and Proceedings,* 27th Leg., 3rd
Sess. (November 26, 2013) (Dustin Duncan, Saskatchewan Party), https://docs.
legassembly.sk.ca/legdocs/Legislative%20Assembly/Hansard/27L3S/131126
Debates.pdf.

15 Ombudsman Saskatchewan, *Caring in Crisis: An Investigation into the Response
to the COVID-19 Outbreak at Extendicare Parkside* (Regina: Ombudsman Saskatchewan, 2021), 58, https://ombudsman.sk.ca/app/uploads/2021/08/Caring
-in-Crisis-Full-Report.pdf.

16 "Third Resident at Extendicare Parkside Dies after Testing Positive for
COVID-19," *CBC News,* December 6, 2020, https://www.cbc.ca/news/canada/
saskatoon/third-resident-at-extendicare-parkside-dies-after-testing-positive
-for-covid-19-1.5830540.

17 Guy Quenneville, "Early Missteps Made Outbreak at Parkside Care Home
Worse, Extendicare Workers Say," *CBC News,* December 16, 2020, https://www.
cbc.ca/news/canada/saskatchewan/extendicare-parkside-regina-care-home
-outbreak-covid-19-1.5840770.

18 David Giles, "Sask. NDP Calls for Public Inquiry into COVID-19 at Extendicare
Parkside," *Global News,* January 14, 2021, https://globalnews.ca/news/7576402/
saskatchewak-ndp-coronavirus-covid-19-outbreak-extendicare-parkside/.

19 Jonathan Guignard, "Saskatchewan Requests Investigation into COVID-19
Outbreak at Regina's Extendicare Parkside," *Global News,* January 29, 2021,
https://globalnews.ca/news/7607821/saskatchewan-covid-19-outbreak-regina
-extendicare-parkside/.

20 Ombudsman Saskatchewan, *Caring in Crisis,* 4.

21 David Shield, "Families of Sask. Extendicare Residents Launch Class-Action
Lawsuit against Care-Home Company," *CBC News,* March 10, 2021, https://
www.cbc.ca/news/canada/saskatchewan/class-action-lawsuit-launched-against
-extendicare-homes-1.5943799.

22 Ombudsman Saskatchewan, *Caring in Crisis,* 58.

23 Ombudsman Saskatchewan, *Caring in Crisis,* 39

24 Quoted in Ombudsman Saskatchewan, *Caring in Crisis,* 59.

25 Ombudsman Saskatchewan, *Caring in Crisis,* 88.

26 Ombudsman Saskatchewan, *Caring in Crisis*, 90.

27 Ombudsman Saskatchewan, *Caring in Crisis*, 28.

28 Ombudsman Saskatchewan, *Caring in Crisis*, 93.

29 Ombudsman Saskatchewan, *Caring in Crisis*, 12.

30 Ombudsman Saskatchewan, *Caring in Crisis*, 94.

31 Ombudsman Saskatchewan, *Caring in Crisis*, 43.

32 Vikram R. Comondore et al., "Quality of Care in For-Profit and Not-for-Profit Nursing Homes: Systematic Review and Meta-Analysis," *BMJ* 339 (August 2009): b2732, https://doi.org/10.1136/bmj.b2732.

33 P.J. Devereaux et al., "Payments for Care at Private For-Profit and Private Not-for-Profit Hospitals: A Systematic Review and Meta-Analysis," *CMAJ* 170, 12 (June 2004): 1817–24, https://doi.org/10.1503/cmaj.1040722.

34 Richard Warnica, "The Problem with Profits: As Ontario's Long-Term-Care Homes Stagger under a COVID Death Toll of More Than 3,000, Some Say It's Time to Shut Down For-Profit Homes for Good," *Toronto Star*, January 26, 2021, https://www.thestar.com/business/2021/01/26/the-problem-with-profits-as-ontarios-long-term-care-homes-stagger-under-a-covid-death-toll-of-more-than-3000-some-say-its-time-to-shut-down-for-profit-homes-for-good.html.

35 Nathan M. Stall et al., "COVID-19 and Ontario's Long-Term Care Homes," *Science Briefs of the Ontario COVID-19 Science Advisory Table* 2, 7 (January 2021): 16, https://covid19-sciencetable.ca/sciencebrief/covid-19-and-ontarios-long-term-care-homes-2/.

36 Stall et al., "COVID-19 and Ontario's Long-Term Care Homes," 12.

37 Adam Hunter, "3 Residents Die following Positive COVID Tests at Regina Care Home," *CBC News*, September 13, 2022, https://www.cbc.ca/news/canada/saskatchewan/regina-elmview-covid-outbreak-1.6581296.

38 Cameron Feil, Natalie Iciaszczyk, and Samir Sinha, *Pandemic Perspectives on Long-Term Care: Insights from Canadians in Light of COVID-19* (Toronto: National Institute on Ageing, 2021), 5, https://www.cma.ca/sites/default/files/pdf/Activities/National-Institute-on-Ageing-CMA-Report-EN.pdf.

39 *A Perfect Storm: The COVID-19 Experience for Revera and the Long Term Care Sector* (Mississauga: Revera, n.d.), https://cdn.reveraliving.com/-/media/files/pandemic-response/expert-advisory-report.pdf.

40 Picard, *Neglected No More*, 178–79.

41 Picard, *Neglected No More*.

42 Picard, *Neglected No More*, 51.

43 Picard, *Neglected No More*, 178.

44 National Institute on Ageing, *Pandemic Perspectives on Long-Term Care*.

45 Picard, *Neglected No More*, 179.

46 Picard, *Neglected No More*, 169.

47 Picard, *Neglected No More*, 169.

48 Picard, *Neglected No More*, 138.

49 Picard, *Neglected No More*, 110.

50 Picard, *Neglected No More*, 110.

Total cases and deaths in Canada from Max Roser, Hannah Ritchie, Esteban Ortiz-Ospina, and Joe Hasell, "Coronavirus Pandemic (COVID-19)," *Our World in Data*, https://ourworldindata.org/coronavirus/country/canada. Total deaths in Saskatchewan from "Saskatchewan's Dashboard – Health and Wellness," Government of Saskatchewan, https://dashboard.saskatchewan. ca/health-wellness.

Miracles and Mudholes

1 "Vaccine Development, Testing, and Regulation," History of Vaccines, College of Physicians of Philadelphia, https://historyofvaccines.org/vaccines-101/how -are-vaccines-made/vaccine-development-testing-and-regulation.

2 Lancet Commission on COVID-19 Vaccines and Therapeutics Task Force Members, "Operation Warp Speed: Implications for Global Vaccine Security," *Lancet Global Health* 9 (March 2021): e1017–e1021, https://doi.org/10.1016/ S2214-109X(21)00140-6.

3 Marc Smith, "Sask. COVID-19 Vaccination Rate Second Highest in Canada," *CTV News*, April 14, 2021, https://regina.ctvnews.ca/sask-covid-19-vaccination -rate-second-highest-in-canada-1.5387334.

4 "Social Contours and COVID-19," Saskatchewan Population Health and Evaluation Research Unit (SPHERU), https://spheru.ca/covid-19/socialcontours/ covid-19-results.php.

5 Mickey Djuric, "Weeks Away from a Full Reopen, Data Shows Sask. Has Lowest Vaccination Rate among Canadian Provinces," *CBC News*, June 23, 2021, https://www.cbc.ca/news/canada/saskatchewan/saskatchewan-lowest -vaccination-rate-among-canadian-province-covid-19-1.6076246.

6 Saskatchewan NDP Caucus, "Meili Calls for 'Last Mile Lottery' to Increase Vaccine Uptake in Saskatchewan," news release, June 7, 2021, https://www. ndpcaucus.sk.ca/meili_calls_for_last_mile_lottery_to_increase_vaccine_ uptake_in_saskatchewan.

7 Djuric, "Weeks Away."

8 "Reported Side Effects following COVID-19 Vaccination in Canada," Government of Canada, updated October 28, 2022, https://health-infobase. canada.ca/covid-19/vaccine-safety/.

9 Mayo Clinic Staff, "Comparing the Differences between COVID-19 Vaccines," Mayo Clinic, October 26, 2022, https://www.mayoclinic.org/coronavirus -covid-19/vaccine/comparing-vaccines.

10 Mayo Clinic Staff, "Comparing the Differences."

11 Rosalie Wyonch and Tingting Zhang, *Damage Averted: Estimating the Effects of Covid-19 Vaccines on Hospitalizations, Mortality and Costs in Canada* (Toronto: C.D. Howe Institute, 2022), https://www.cdhowe.org/public-policy-research/ damage-averted-estimating-effects-covid-19-vaccines-hospitalizations.

12 Government of Saskatchewan, "Influenza Cases in Saskatchewan, Get Your Flu Shot Today," news release, November 15, 2022, https://www.saskatchewan.ca/government/news-and-media/2022/november/15/influenza-cases-in-saskatchewan-get-your-flu-shot-today.

13 Government of Saskatchewan, "Protecting Saskatchewan Residents from Influenza: 295,165 Flu Shots Administered in Two Months," news release, December 8, 2021, https://www.saskatchewan.ca/government/news-and-media/2021/december/08/protecting-saskatchewan-residents-from-influenza-295165-flu-shots-administered-in-2-months.

14 Alessia Passafiume, "Flu Vaccine Uptake for Canadians 'Stubbornly Low,' Older Canadians Not Meeting Targets," *Toronto Star*, November 29, 2022, https://www.thestar.com/news/canada/2022/11/29/flu-vaccine-uptake-for-canadians-stubbornly-low-older-canadians-not-meeting-targets.html.

15 Carly Weeks, "Routine Vaccination Rates for Children, Teens in Canada Dropped Dramatically since Start of COVID-19 Pandemic," *Globe and Mail*, August 30, 2022, https://www.theglobeandmail.com/canada/article-routine-vaccination-rates-children-teens.

16 "24 Confirmed Whooping Cough Cases in Southern Alberta Outbreak," *CBC News*, February 2, 2023, https://www.cbc.ca/news/canada/calgary/whooping-cough-cases-southern-alberta-outbreak-1.6735125.

17 Weeks, "Routine Vaccination Rates."

18 Stephanie Dubois, "What We Know about Why Some Kids Are Missing Routine Vaccinations," *CBC News*, August 19, 2022, https://www.cbc.ca/news/health/kids-missing-routine-vaccinations-1.6555077.

19 Natalie Iciaszczyk et al., *A Goal within Our Reach: What the COVID-19 Pandemic Has Taught Us about Improving the Uptake of Influenza Vaccinations in Canada* (Toronto: National Institute on Ageing, 2022), https://static1.squarespace.com/static/5c2fa7b03917eed9b5a436d8/t/6385fbf18cd7a156622addc7/1669725171981/Final+Report+-+A+Goal+Within+Our+Reach+-+Influenza+Vaccination2+.pdf.

20 Chris Beyrer, "The Long History of mRNA Vaccines," Johns Hopkins, Bloomberg School of Public Health, October 6, 2021, https://publichealth.jhu.edu/2021/the-long-history-of-mrna-vaccines.

21 SciDev.Net, "Hunting the 'Perfect Protein' for Malaria mRNA Vaccine," VaccinesWork, April 25, 2022, https://www.gavi.org/vaccineswork/hunting-perfect-protein-malaria-mrna-vaccine; Jennifer Abbasi, "First mRNA HIV Vaccine Clinical Trial Launches," *JAMA* 327, 10 (2022): 909.

22 Edward Winstead, "Can mRNA Vaccines Help Treat Cancer?" National Cancer Institute, January 20, 2022, https://www.cancer.gov/news-events/cancer-currents-blog/2022/mrna-vaccines-to-treat-cancer.

23 Sam Maciag, "Sask. Vaccine Manufacturing Facility the First of Its Kind in Canada," *CBC News*, June 28, 2022, https://www.cbc.ca/news/canada/saskatchewansask-vaccine-manufacturing-facility-first-of-kind-in-canada-1.6503798.

1   Guy Quenneville and Adam Hunter, "Emotional Premier Moe Talks 'Most Difficult' Pandemic Decisions in Sask.," *CBC News*, May 12, 2021, https://www. cbc.ca/news/canada/saskatoon/covid-19-scott-moe-emotional-pandemic-may -2021-1.6024405.

2   Derek Ruttle, "Premier Moe, MLA Skoropad Hear from Public in Town Hall Forum," *SaskToday.ca*, July 11, 2022, https://www.sasktoday.ca/central/outlook/ premier-moe-mla-skoropad-hear-from-public-in-town-hall-forum-5571845.

3   Arthur White-Crummey, "Meili Challenges Moe to Visit ICU, but Premier Says 'Inappropriate,'" *Regina Leader-Post*, April 19, 2021, https://leaderpost.com/ news/saskatchewan/meili-challenges-moe-to-visit-icu-but-premier-says -inappropriate.

4   "Regina Critical Care Lead Would Welcome ICU Visit from Premier Moe," *CBC News*, April 26, 2021, https://www.cbc.ca/news/canada/saskatoon/ regina-critical-care-lead-would-welcome-icu-visit-from-premier-moe-1. 6001746.

5   Jörg Broschek, "Federalism, Political Leadership and the COVID-19 Pandemic: Explaining Canada's Tale of Two Federations," *Territory, Politics, Governance* 10, 6 (2022): 779–98, https://doi.org/10.1080/21622671.2022.2101513.

6   Broschek, "Federalism, Political Leadership."

7   Julie Gordon, "Canada's Atlantic Region Closed Out World to Beat COVID-19, and the Economy Has Done OK," *Reuters*, October 25, 2020, https://www. reuters.com/article/us-health-coronavirus-canada-economy-idUKKBN 27A0KG.

8   Andrew Nikiforuk, "Canada Is One Big Pandemic Response Experiment. It Proves 'Zero COVID' Is Best," *The Tyee*, April 2, 2021, https://thetyee.ca/ News/2021/04/02/Canada-One-Big-Pandemic-Response-Experiment -Zero-COVID.

9   Chris Hall, "'I'll Do Whatever I Have To': N.S. Premier Iain Rankin Doubles Down on Lockdown," *CBC News*, May 15, 2021, https://www.cbc.ca/radio/ thehouse/iain-rankin-pandemic-nova-scotia-covid-lockdown-1.6017785.

10 Phil Tank, "Phil Tank: Saskatchewan Lays Out Welcome Mat for Latest COVID-19 Wave," *Saskatoon StarPhoenix*, October 20, 2022, https://thestar phoenix.com/opinion/columnists/phil-tank-saskatchewan-lays-out-welcome -mat-for-latest-covid-19-wave.

11 Emily Cameron-Blake et al., "Variation in the Canadian Provincial and Ter- ritorial Responses to COVID-19" (working paper, Blavatnik School of Gov- ernment, University of Oxford, March 2021), 28, https://www.bsg.ox.ac.uk/ sites/default/files/2021-03/BSG-WP-2021-039.pdf.

12 Andrew M. Morris and Jack M. Mintz, "A 'No More Waves' Strategy for COVID-19 in Canada," *CMAJ* 193, 4 (2021): 132–34, https://www.cmaj.ca/ content/cmaj/193/4/E132.full.pdf; Roberto Rocha, Inayat Singh, and Julianna Perkins, "Provinces That Acted Faster Had More Success at Limiting Spread of COVID-19, Data Suggests," *CBC News*, December 26, 2020, https://www. cbc.ca/news/canada/stringency-covid-lockdown-wave-1.5853785; COVID

Strategic Choices Group, *Building the Canadian Shield: A New Strategy to Protect Canadians from COVID and from the Fight against COVID* (December 30, 2020), https://jdi.queensu.ca/wp-content/uploads/2021/04/Building-the-Canadian-Shield.pdf.

13 Adam Hunter, "Meili Calls Moe's Lockdown Comment 'Slap in the Face' to Health-Care Workers and Those Grieving, Sick," *CBC News*, February 9, 2021, https://www.cbc.ca/news/canada/saskatchewan/meili-moe-lockdown-1.5906945?__vfz=medium%3Dsharebar.

14 CPAC, "Saskatchewan Update on COVID-19 – February 25, 2021," video, 50:54, February 25, 2021, https://www.youtube.com/watch?v=R6mbEQ5jo_g.

15 Saskatchewan Health Authority, "Physician Town Hall," presentation, March 18, 2021.

16 Arthur White-Crummey, "COVID-19: Bubbles Can Grow to 10 in Saskatchewan, 35 Variant Cases Detected," *Regina Leader-Post*, March 9, 2021, https://leaderpost.com/news/saskatchewan/covid-19-bubbles-can-grow-to-10-in-saskatchewan-35-variant-cases-detected.

17 Zak Vescera, "Emails Hint at Divide between Shahab, Government on COVID-19 in 2021," *Saskatoon StarPhoenix*, July 7, 2022, https://thestarphoenix.com/news/saskatchewan/emails-hint-at-divide-between-shahab-government-on-covid-19-in-2021.

18 Kendall Latimer, "Mom Pleads for People to Take COVID Seriously as Her Son Fights for His Life in Regina ICU," *CBC News*, March 31, 2021, https://www.cbc.ca/news/canada/saskatchewan/regina-34-year-old-covid-icu-1.5969837?__vfz=medium%3Dsharebar.

19 Zak Vescera, "The Virus Changed. Should Saskatchewan's Vaccine Plan Do the Same?" *Saskatoon StarPhoenix*, April 6, 2021, https://thestarphoenix.com/news/saskatchewan/the-virus-changed-should-saskatchewans-vaccine-plan-do-the-same.

20 Kendall Latimer, "Sask. Man Calls on Province to Tweak Vaccination Priorities after Close Call with COVID," *CBC News*, April 8, 2021, https://www.cbc.ca/news/canada/saskatchewan/matthew-cardinal-covid-recovery-1.5978554.

21 Alina S. Schnake-Mahl et al., "Higher COVID-19 Vaccination and Narrower Disparities in US Cities with Paid Sick Leave Compared to Those Without," *Health Affairs* 41, 11 (2022): 1565–74, https://doi.org/10.1377/hlthaff.2022.00779.

22 Office of the Premier, Government of British Columbia, "Five Paid Sick Days Coming Jan. 1," news release, November 24, 2021, https://news.gov.bc.ca/releases/2021PREM0073-002235.

23 Colleen Silverthorn, "Regina Father Dies of COVID-19 Days after Couple's 3rd Child Is Born," *CBC News*, April 26, 2021, https://www.cbc.ca/news/canada/saskatchewan/regina-father-dies-covid-19-1.6002267.

24 "Home," Fight for $15, https://fightfor15.org/.

25 Kendall Latimer, "Sask. People Struggling to Make Ends Meet on Minimum Wage," *CBC News*, March 7, 2022, https://www.cbc.ca/news/canada/saskatoon/sask-minimum-wage-cost-of-living-1.6370454.

26 Canadian Centre for Policy Alternatives, "A Living Wage for Regina Is $16.23/Hour, Saskatoon Is $16.89 Per Hour: Report," news release, May 27, 2022,

https://policyalternatives.ca/newsroom/news-releases/living-wage-regina
-1623hour-saskatoon-1689-hour-report.

FOURTH WAVE

Total cases and deaths in Canada from Max Roser, Hannah Ritchie, Esteban
Ortiz-Ospina, and Joe Hasell, "Coronavirus Pandemic (COVID-19)," *Our
World in Data*, https://ourworldindata.org/coronavirus/country/canada. Total
deaths in Saskatchewan from "Saskatchewan's Dashboard – Health and
Wellness," Government of Saskatchewan, https://dashboard.saskatchewan.
ca/health-wellness.

Best Summer Ever

1 Alexander Quon, "Handshake Seals Final Regular COVID-19 Update as
  Sask. Issues Guidance for 3rd Phase of Reopening," *CBC News*, July 7, 2021,
  https://www.cbc.ca/news/canada/saskatchewan/sask-covid-19-reopening-1.
  6093677.
2 Arthur White-Crummey, "Moe Says Cautious Federal Reopening Advice
  Won't Slow Down Sask.," *Regina Leader-Post*, May 14, 2021, https://leaderpost.
  com/news/saskatchewan/moe-says-cautious-federal-reopening-advice-wont
  -slow-down-sask.
3 Scott Moe (@PremierScottMoe), "The good news is – Saskatchewan won't be
  following the federal plan ...," Twitter, May 14, 2021, https://twitter.com/premier
  scottmoe/status/1393323045868097540?lang=en.
4 Alex Boyd, "Jason Kenney Lays Out Plan for 'the Best Alberta Summer Ever'
  – with COVID Reopening That Outpaces Ontario," *Toronto Star*, May 26, 2021,
  https://www.thestar.com/news/canada/2021/05/26/weeks-after-facing-north
  -americas-highest-covid-rates-alberta-unveils-plan-to-almost-fully-reopen-by
  -early-july.html.
5 Jason Kenney, "Congratulations to my friend Premier Scott Moe ...," Facebook, July 12, 2021, https://www.facebook.com/kenneyjasont/photos/a.
  10153076743492641/10159343008112641/?type=3.
6 Yasmine Ghania, "'Fall and Winter of Misery': Sask.'s Top Doctor Says There
  May Not Be Large Thanksgiving, Christmas Gatherings," *CBC News*, September 29, 2021, https://www.cbc.ca/news/canada/saskatchewan/health
  -minister-paul-merriman-shahab-covid-vaccine-1.6194242.
7 Zak Vescera, "How the Fourth Wave of COVID-19 Beat Saskatchewan,"
  Saskatoon StarPhoenix, September 16, 2021, https://thestarphoenix.com/news/
  saskatchewan/how-the-fourth-wave-of-covid-19-beat-saskatchewan.
8 Zak Vescera, "COVID-19: Why Is Saskatchewan's Vaccination Rate So Low?"
  Saskatoon StarPhoenix, October 15, 2021, https://thestarphoenix.com/news/
  local-news/covid-19-why-is-saskatchewans-vaccination-rate-so-low.
9 Guy Quenneville, "Newly Shared Sask. COVID-19 Modelling from June
  Projected This Fall's Surge of ICU Patients," *CBC News*, October 26, 2021,
  https://www.cbc.ca/news/canada/saskatoon/covid-19-modelling-1.6224092.

10 Quenneville, "Newly Shared Sask. COVID-19 Modelling."

11 Saskatchewan Health Authority, "Physician Town Hall," presentation, October 21, 2021, https://www.saskhealthauthority.ca/system/files/2022-06/Presentation-PSA-Physician-Town-Hall-October-21-2021.pdf.

12 Cory Coleman, "Sask. Opposition NDP, Federation of Labour Call for COVID-19 Mandates, Health Minister to Resign," *CBC News*, August 30, 2021, https://www.cbc.ca/news/canada/saskatchewan/covid-19-mandates-resignation-1.6158710.

13 Bryan Eneas, "Sask. Doctors Warned by Public Health Officials That More Measures Are Necessary to Blunt 4th Wave," *CBC News*, August 27, 2021, https://www.cbc.ca/lite/story/1.6155828.

14 Guy Quenneville, "Sask. Doctors Ask Gov't for Vaccine Passports and Other 4th Wave Measures, Moe Nixes 'Heavy-Handed' Approach," *CBC News*, August 30, 2021, https://www.cbc.ca/news/canada/saskatoon/cory-neudorf-saskatchewan-health-authority-medical-health-officers-letter-covid-19-fourth-wave-1.6158503.

15 Quenneville, "Sask. Doctors Ask Gov't for Vaccine Passports."

16 Alexander Quon, "Premier Scott Moe Admits Sask. Could Have Responded Faster to 4th Wave of COVID-19," *CBC News*, October 19, 2021, https://www.cbc.ca/news/canada/saskatchewan/premier-moe-admits-could-have-responded-faster-to-4th-wave-1.6216535.

17 World Health Organization, "UNODC, WHO, UNAIDS and OHCHR Joint Statement on COVID-19 in Prisons and Other Closed Settings," public statement, May 13, 2020, https://www.who.int/news/item/13-05-2020-unodc-who-unaids-and-ohchr-joint-statement-on-covid-19-in-prisons-and-other-closed-settings.

18 Dan Zakreski, "Province-Wide Group Calls for Massive Release of Sask. Prisoners to Stop Spread of COVID-19," *CBC News*, April 3, 2020, https://www.cbc.ca/news/canada/saskatoon/provice-wide-group-calls-for-release-of-prisoners-1.5520726.

19 Stephanie Taylor, "Corrections Minister Won't Pursue How COVID-19 Spread in Saskatoon Jail," *Toronto Star*, December 1, 2020, https://www.thestar.com/news/canada/2020/12/01/more-than-100-inmates-23-staff-test-positive-for-covid-19-at-saskatoon-jail.html.

20 Taylor, "Corrections Minister Won't Pursue."

21 Cory Cardinal, "'Tomorrow We Take Action': How Sask. Inmates Rallied for Safer Conditions during the Pandemic," *CBC News*, February 1, 2021, https://www.cbc.ca/news/canada/saskatoon/pov-cory-cardinal-inmates-rallied-pandemic-1.5894078.

22 Dan Zakreski, "Inmates in Saskatoon, Prince Albert Stage Hunger Strike and Call for Resignation of Christine Tell," *CBC News*, January 4, 2021, https://www.cbc.ca/news/canada/saskatoon/inmates-in-saskatoon-prince-albert-stage-hunger-strike-1.5860712.

23 Cardinal, "'Tomorrow We Take Action.'"

24 Morgan Modjeski, "Families, Opposition Want Sask. Inmates Prioritized for Vaccines as Outbreaks Continue," *CBC News*, April 24, 2021, https://www.cbc.

ca/news/canada/saskatoon/families-opposition-want-sask-inmates-prioritized
-for-vaccines-as-outbreaks-continue-1.6001132.

25 Morgan Modjeski, "Sister Says Kimberly Squirrel Not Dressed for Sask. Winter
after Release from Provincial Jail," *CBC News*, February 22, 2021, https://www.
cbc.ca/news/canada/saskatoon/kimberly-squirrel-follow-1.5922456.

26 Thia James, "Life Cut Short for Cory Charles Cardinal, Sask. Advocate for the
Incarcerated," *Saskatoon StarPhoenix*, June 11, 2021, https://thestarphoenix.com/
news/local-news/life-cut-short-for-cory-charles-cardinal-sask-advocate-for
-the-incarcerated.

27 Zak Vescera, "Sask. Government Knows Safe Consumption Sites Save Lives
– but Won't Fund Them," *Saskatoon StarPhoenix*, April 10, 2021, https://
thestarphoenix.com/news/saskatchewan/in-saskatchewan-a-battle-over
-supervised-drug-use.

28 Vescera, "Sask. Government Knows Safe Consumption Sites Save Lives."

29 Bryan Eneas, "Public Perception Shifting as Sask. Overdoses Numbers Climb
in 2021: Prairie Harm Reduction Executive Director," *CBC News*, December
26, 2021, https://www.cbc.ca/news/canada/saskatoon/prairie-harm-reduction
-2021-year-ender-1.6298531.

30 Morgan Modjeski, "Sask. Writer, Poet, and Prisoner Advocate Cory Cardinal
Dead at 38," *CBC News*, June 11, 2021, https://www.cbc.ca/news/canada/
saskatoon/cory-cardinal-file-1-1.6062737.

31 Modjeski, "Sask. Writer, Poet, and Prisoner Advocate Cory Cardinal Dead
at 38."

32 Government of Canada, "Opioid and Stimulant-Related Harms in Canada,"
Health Infobase, September 2022, https://health-infobase.canada.ca/substance-
related-harms/opioids-stimulants/.

33 Theresa Kliem, "Sask. Could See Even More Overdose Deaths This Year Than
in 2021, Report Suggests," *CBC News*, September 10, 2022, https://www.cbc.
ca/news/canada/saskatchewan/overdose-deaths-saskatchewan-2022-august
-31-1.6578398.

The Dam Breaks

1 Laura Sciarpelletti, "'I Feel Betrayed by My Government': Resident, NDP
Call on Sask. to Resume Organ Donor Program," *CBC News*, November 8,
2021, https://www.cbc.ca/news/canada/saskatchewan/ndp-official-opposition
-call-on-sask-government-to-resume-organ-donor-program-1.6241786.

2 Connor O'Donovan, "'27 Missed Opportunities' for Organ Donations with
Program Paused: SHA," *Global News*, November 8, 2021, https://globalnews.ca/
news/8358556/missed-opportunities-organ-donations-program-paused-sha/.

3 Nathaniel Dove, "Saskatchewan Organ Transplant Patients Still Waiting for
Surgeries," *Global News*, March 15, 2022, https://globalnews.ca/news/8685839/
saskatchewan-organ-transplant-patients-surgeries/.

4 Alec Salloum, "'I'm Getting Sicker and Sicker Every Day:' Woman Calls on
Government to Tackle Mounting Backlog of Surgeries," *Regina Leader-*

Post, November 29, 2021, https://leaderpost.com/news/politics/surgery-wait
-times.

5   Arthur White-Crummey, "Moe Says Organ Program Resuming by Month's
    End, but Wait Horrifies Patient," *Regina Leader-Post*, November 17, 2021, https://
    leaderpost.com/news/saskatchewan/moe-says-organ-program-resuming-by
    -months-end-but-wait-horrifies-patient.

6   Arthur White-Crummey, "'This Is a Priority,' Moe Tells Woman Ailing from
    Hip Surgery Delay," *Regina Leader-Post*, November 4, 2021, https://leaderpost.
    com/news/saskatchewan/this-is-a-priority-moe-tells-woman-ailing-from
    -hip-surgery-delay.

7   Arthur White-Crummey, "Toddler with Spina Bifida Another Lesson for
    Health Minister," *Regina Leader-Post*, November 18, 2021, https://leaderpost.
    com/news/saskatchewan/toddler-with-spina-bifida-another-lesson-for
    -health-minister.

8   Zak Vescera, "Sask. Modelling Says Masks Could Reduce Infections by Up to
    50 Per Cent," *Saskatoon StarPhoenix*, September 10, 2021, https://thestarphoenix.
    com/news/local-news/sask-modelling-says-masks-could-reduce-infections-by
    -up-to-50-per-cent.

9   Vescera, "Sask. Modelling."

10 "Moe Says Unvaccinated Will Find Things 'More Uncomfortable' in Sask.,"
    650 CKOM, August 30, 2021, https://www.ckom.com/2021/08/30/moe
    -says-unvaccinated-will-find-things-more-uncomfortable-in-sask/.

11 Nathaniel Dove, "Saskatchewan Government Emails Warned of Health-Care
    Collapse ahead of COVID Patient Transfer," *Global News*, March 17, 2023,
    https://globalnews.ca/news/9559647/sask-govt-emails-health-care-collapse
    -covid-patient-transfer/.

12 Zak Vescera, "Sask. to Cancel Many Elective Surgeries; Must Bargain with
    Unions on Staff Redeployment," *Saskatoon StarPhoenix*, September 10, 2021,
    https://thestarphoenix.com/news/local-news/sask-to-cancel-many-elective
    -surgeries-must-bargain-with-unions-on-staff-redeployment.

13 "Saskatoon ICU Doctor Says Organ Donation Suspension Is 'Just the
    Beginning' amid Surging COVID-19 Cases," *CTV News*, September 24, 2021,
    https://saskatoon.ctvnews.ca/saskatoon-icu-doctor-says-organ-donation
    -suspension-is-just-the-beginning-amid-surging-covid-19-cases-1.5599861.

14 Adam Hunter, "Sask. Premier Scott Moe Announces Mandatory Masking and
    Proof of Vaccination Policies," *CBC News*, September 16, 2021, https://www.
    cbc.ca/news/canada/saskatchewan/sask-covid-update-moe-1.6178096.

15 Adam Hunter, "Sask. Premier's Messaging Diverges from Health-Care Offi-
    cials amid Refusal to Adopt COVID-19 Restrictions," *CBC News*, October 9,
    2021, https://www.cbc.ca/news/canada/saskatchewan/sask-covid-19-fourth
    -wave-1.6204791.

16 "Alberta to Launch Proof-of-Vaccination Program, Declares Health Emergency
    amid Surge in COVID-19 Cases," *CBC News*, September 15, 2021, https://www.
    cbc.ca/news/canada/edmonton/kenney-shandro-hinshaw-update-covid-19-1.
    6177210.

17 Jason Warick, "Inaccurate, Unfair for Sask. Premier to Single Out Northern First Nations on Vaccination, Say Critics," *CBC News,* September 24, 2021, https://www.cbc.ca/news/canada/saskatoon/northern-first-nations-covid -19-scott-moe-1.6187634.

18 Adam Hunter, "Moe Says No to Vaccine Mandates, Passports but Expects Businesses, Organizations Will Enact Policies," *CBC News,* August 27, 2021, https://www.cbc.ca/news/canada/saskatchewan/sask-vaccine-mandate-1. 6155047.

19 Zak Vescera, "COVID-19: Why Is Saskatchewan's Vaccination Rate So Low?" *Saskatoon StarPhoenix,* October 15, 2021, https://thestarphoenix.com/news/ local-news/covid-19-why-is-saskatchewans-vaccination-rate-so-low.

20 Adam Hunter, "Trudeau Criticizes Moe as Sask. Sets COVID-19 Case Record, Trails 8 Provinces in Shots," *CBC News,* September 14, 2021, https://www.cbc. ca/news/canada/saskatchewan/sask-covid-trudeau-moe-1.6175081.

21 Katharine Smart, "We Need to Mobilize Now: Alberta and Saskatchewan's Health Systems at Breaking Point," news release, Canadian Medical Association, September 29, 2021, https://www.cma.ca/news-releases-and-statements/ we-need-mobilize-now-alberta-and-saskatchewans-health-systems-breaking.

22 Smart, "We Need to Mobilize Now."

23 Dayne Patterson, "Deputy Chief Says Saskatoon Police Should Have Recommended that PPC Election Event Be Cancelled," *CBC News,* September 29, 2021, https://www.cbc.ca/news/canada/saskatchewan/ppc-election-event -saskatoon-hotel-police-tickets-fines-citations-1.6194132.

24 Mack Lamoreux, "Anti-Vax Influencer and Failed Politician Now Intubated in ICU for COVID," *Vice,* October 25, 2021, https://www.vice.com/en/article/ akvw9b/mark-friesen-anti-vax-canadian-politician-intubated-covid.

25 "COVID-19 in Sask.: Canadian Military Leaves Province as Active Cases Decrease," *CBC News,* December 5, 2021, https://www.cbc.ca/news/canada/ saskatchewan/covid-19-sask-dec-5-canadian-military-leaves-saskatchewan-1. 6274448.

26 Alexander Quon, "Premier Scott Moe Admits Sask. Could Have Responded Faster to 4th Wave of COVID-19," *CBC News,* October 19, 2021, https://www. cbc.ca/news/canada/saskatchewan/premier-moe-admits-could-have-responded -faster-to-4th-wave-1.6216535.

27 Guy Quenneville, "Chief Medical Health Officer Says Sask. Gov't Needs to Look at Expanding Reach of COVID Measures," *CBC News,* October 25, 2021, https://www.cbc.ca/news/canada/saskatoon/dr-saqib-shahab-covid-19 -recommendations-saskatchewan-government-1.6224107.

28 Adam Hunter, "Sask. Premier Says Additional Health Measures Not Fair to Those Who Have Been Vaccinated," *CBC News,* October 25, 2021, https://www. cbc.ca/news/canada/saskatchewan/scott-moe-address-sask-health-1.6224029.

29 Saskatchewan Health Authority, "Physician Town Hall," presentation, October 21, 2021, https://www.saskhealthauthority.ca/system/files/2022-06/Presentation -PSA-Physician-Town-Hall-October-21-2021.pdf.

30 Michael Warner (@drmwarner), Twitter, October 20, 2021, https://twitter.com/ drmwarner/status/1450891996189626374.

31 Yasmine Ghania, "6 Saskatchewan ICU Patients with COIVD-19 Being Transferred to Ontario," *CBC News,* October 18, 2021, https://www.cbc.ca/news/canada/saskatchewan/ontario-covid-icu-patients-transfer-1.6215022.

32 Bryn Levy, "Sask. Doctor Reports Further Patient Transfers to Ontario Halted," *Saskatoon StarPhoenix,* October 20, 2021, https://thestarphoenix.com/news/local-news/sask-doctor-reports-further-patient-transfers-to-ontario-halted.

33 Levy, "Sask. Doctor Reports Further Patient Transfers to Ontario Halted."

34 Bonnie Allen, "Sask. COVID-19 Patient Marks 279 days in Hospital," *CBC News,* April 29, 2022, https://www.cbc.ca/news/canada/saskatoon/sask-covid-19-patient-marks-279-days-in-hospital-1.6436453.

35 Alexander Quon and Jessie Anton, "Dr. Shahab Says Pleas from Health Officers in Line with His Own Recommendations to Government," *CBC News,* October 26, 2021, https://www.cbc.ca/news/canada/saskatchewan/dr-shahab-says-pleas-from-health-officers-in-line-with-his-own-recommendations-to-government-1.6225248.

36 Quon and Anton, "Dr. Shahab Says Pleas."

37 Quon and Anton, "Dr. Shahab Says Pleas."

38 Murray Mandryk, "Mandryk: Livingstone Departure May Be Foreshadowing Bigger Problem," *Regina Leader-Post,* December 4, 2021, https://leaderpost.com/opinion/columnists/mandryk-livingstone-departure-may-be-foreshadowing-bigger-problem.

39 Yasmine Ghania, "Sask. Schools Shouldn't Exclude Unvaccinated Students from Extracurricular Activities: Education Minister," *CBC News,* November 17, 2021, https://www.cbc.ca/news/canada/saskatchewan/schools-exracurricular-school-unvaccinated-students-covid-1.6253002.

40 Wayne Mantyka, "Parents Must Now Be Present for COVD-19 Vaccinations in Sask. Elementary Schools," *CTV News,* November 30, 2021, https://regina.ctvnews.ca/parents-must-now-be-present-for-covid-19-vaccinations-in-sask-elementary-schools-1.5688162.

41 "COVID-19 Vaccination in Canada," Government of Canada, updated October 9, 2022, https://health-infobase.canada.ca/covid-19/vaccination-coverage/.

42 Hunter, "Sask. Premier's Messaging Diverges from Health-Care Officials."

43 Hunter, "Sask. Premier's Messaging Diverges from Health-Care Officials."

44 Cory Coleman, "Sask. Health Authority CEO Scott Livingstone Resigns from Position, Effective Immediately," *CBC News,* December 2, 2021, https://www.cbc.ca/news/canada/saskatchewan/scott-livingstone-leaves-position-1.6271057.

45 Zak Vescera, "Sask. Party Political Operative Raynelle Wilson Named to Highest Ranks of SHA," *Saskatoon StarPhoenix,* January 14, 2022, https://thestarphoenix.com/news/saskatchewan/sask-party-political-operative-raynelle-wilson-named-to-highest-ranks-of-sha.

46 Zak Vescera, "Numbers Tell the Story of Saskatchewan's Surgery Backlog," *Saskatoon StarPhoenix,* April 27, 2022, https://thestarphoenix.com/news/saskatchewan/numbers-tell-the-story-of-saskatchewans-surgery-backlog.

47 "Doctors Call for Reforms as People in Sask. Struggle to Find a Family Doctor," *CBC News,* October 5, 2022, https://www.cbc.ca/news/canada/saskatchewan/doctor-shortage-sask-family-physician-1.6607146.

48 Patrick Rail, "Canada's Health-Care System Is 'Collapsing around Us,' Warns CMA President," *CTV News*, June 15, 2022, https://beta.ctvnews.ca/national/health/2022/6/15/1_5948416.amp.html.

49 Jeremy Nuttall, "Health Ministers' Meeting Ends without Funding Deal as Liberals' Duclos Rips Premiers' 'Marching Orders,'" *Toronto Star*, November 8, 2022, https://www.thestar.com/news/canada/2022/11/08/health-ministers-meeting-ends-without-funding-deal.html.

50 David Macdonald, "No Strings Attached," *The Monitor*, February 15, 2023, https://monitormag.ca/reports/no-strings-attached/.

51 Mickey Djuric, "Saskatchewan to Privatize Some Surgeries to Reduce Growing Backlog from COVID-19," *Globe and Mail*, December 9, 2021, https://www.theglobeandmail.com/canada/article-saskatchewan-to-privatize-some-surgeries-to-reduce-growing-backlog/.

52 Don Braid, "Braid: Smith's Health Spending Accounts Aim at Grooming the Public for Private Payment," *Calgary Herald*, November 21, 2022, https://calgaryherald.com/opinion/columnists/braid-smiths-health-spending-accounts-aim-at-grooming-the-public-for-private-payment.

FIFTH WAVE

Total cases and deaths in Canada from Max Roser, Hannah Ritchie, Esteban Ortiz-Ospina, and Joe Hasell, "Coronavirus Pandemic (COVID-19)," *Our World in Data*, https://ourworldindata.org/coronavirus/country/canada. Total deaths in Saskatchewan from "Saskatchewan's Dashboard – Health and Wellness," Government of Saskatchewan, https://dashboard.saskatchewan.ca/health-wellness.

Putting It Mildly

1 Scott Moe (@PremierScottMoe), "Today, trucker rallies are being held at many locations across the country, including on Parliament Hill in Ottawa and in various communities in Saskatchewan …," Twitter, January 29, 2022, https://twitter.com/premierscottmoe/status/1487460075102871554.

2 Guy Quenneville, "'We're Not Asking You to Storm the Beaches of Normandy,' Sask. Premier Tells Vaccination Holdouts," *CBC News*, May 26, 2021, https://www.cbc.ca/news/canada/saskatoon/saskatchewan-covid-19-vaccine-doubt-normany-second-world-war-premier-scott-moe-1.6040052.

3 Adam Hunter, "Sask. Premier Scott Moe Announces Mandatory Masking and Proof of Vaccination Policies," *CBC News*, September 16, 2021, https://www.cbc.ca/news/canada/saskatchewan/sask-covid-update-moe-1.6178096.

4 Scott Moe (@PremierScottMoe), "Believing in and spreading anti-vaccine conspiracy theories is contributing to people dying from COVID-19 by keeping them from getting vaccinated …," Twitter, October 7, 2021, https://twitter.com/PremierScottMoe/status/1446261075876397060?s=20&t=pe1eiwcfdGTO4UpUvIkk-Q.

5   Noor Ibrahim, "COVID-19: Can Doctors Refuse Unvaccinated Patients? Reports Suggest This Is Already Happening," *Global News*, November 8, 2021, https://globalnews.ca/news/8286334/covid-19-can-doctors-deny-medical-care-to-unvaccineded-patients/.

6   Adam Hunter, "How Sask. Premier Moe's Messaging on Unvaccinated People Has Shifted since the Delta Wave," *CBC News*, February 12, 2022, https://www.cbc.ca/news/canada/saskatchewan/sask-covid-measures-1.6345397.

7   Janet French, "New Alberta Premier Says Unvaccinated 'Most Discriminated against Group' after Swearing-In," *CBC News*, October 11, 2022, https://www.cbc.ca/news/canada/edmonton/new-alberta-premier-says-unvaccinated-most-discriminated-against-group-after-swearing-in-1.6612767.

8   Phil Tank, "Tank: Unified Grassroots Sounds Less about Unity the Closer You Listen," *Saskatoon StarPhoenix*, January 6, 2022, https://thestarphoenix.com/opinion/columnists/tank-unified-grassroots-sounds-less-about-unity-the-closer-you-listen.

9   Emily Leedham, "Group That Had Hour-Long Phone Call with Scott Moe Has Quiet Links to Far-Right Conspiracies," *PressProgress*, January 26, 2022, https://pressprogress.ca/group-that-had-hour-long-phone-call-with-scott-moe-has-quiet-links-to-far-right-conspiracies/.

10 Phil Tank, "Moe Says 'Ridiculous' COVID-19 Conspiracy Theories Costing Sask. Lives," *Saskatoon StarPhoenix*, October 7, 2021, https://thestarphoenix.com/news/local-news/moe-says-ridiculous-covid-19-conspiracy-theories-costing-sask-lives.

11 Darren Major, "COVID-19 Misinformation Cost at Least 2,800 Lives and $300M, New Report Says," *CBC News*, January 27, 2023, https://www.cbc.ca/news/politics/cost-of-covid-19-misinformation-study-1.6726356.

12 Saskatchewan NDP Caucus, "NDP: Expand Booster Shot Eligibility to Protect from Omicron and Prevent 5th Wave," news release, December 3, 2021, https://www.ndpcaucus.sk.ca/ndp_expand_booster_shot_eligibility_to_protect_from_omicron_and_prevent_5th_wave.

13 Scott Moe (@PremierScottMoe), "Is it time to end COVID-19 restrictions? Here's what I think, and what I'm hearing from Saskatchewan people," Twitter, February 2, 2022, https://twitter.com/PremierScottMoe/status/1489045180745494529.

14 Dan Gardner, "Getting Used to Covid," *PastPresentFuture*, March 12, 2022, https://dgardner.substack.com/p/getting-used-to-covid?s=r&utm_campaign=post&utm_medium=web.

15 Jacob Steere-Williams, "Endemic Fatalism and Why It Won't Resolve COVID-19," *BMJ Blog: Medical Humanities*, February 8, 2022, https://blogs.bmj.com/medical-humanities/2022/02/08/endemic-fatalism-and-why-it-wont-resolve-covid-19/.

16 André Picard, "Lessons from Two Years of Pandemic Living," *Globe and Mail*, March 11, 2022, https://www.theglobeandmail.com/canada/article-lessons-from-two-years-of-pandemic-living/.

17 Carrie Tait, "Saskatchewan Premier Scott Moe Won't Bring Back Restrictions to Contain Omicron Spread," *Globe and Mail*, January 12, 2022, https://

www.theglobeandmail.com/canada/article-saskatchewan-premier-scott-moe-to-not-interfere-with-restrictions-to/.

18   Ian Gustafson, "Saskatchewan Nurses Disappointed, Tired amid Province's Fifth Wave of COVID-19," *650 CKOM,* January 13, 2022, https://www.ckom.com/2022/01/13/saskatchewan-nurses-disappointed-tired-amid-provinces-fifth-wave-of-covid-19/.

19   Saskatchewan Health Authority, "Physician Town Hall," presentation, January 27, 2022, https://www.saskhealthauthority.ca/system/files/2022-06/Presentation-PSA-Physician-Town-Hall-January-27-2022.pdf.

20   Murray Mandryk, "Moe's Decision to Remove COVID-19 Restrictions Doesn't Add Up," *Saskatoon StarPhoenix,* January 29, 2022, https://thestarphoenix.com/opinion/columnists/mandryk-moes-decision-to-remove-covid-19-restrictions-doesnt-add-up/wcm/622887d0-4e84-4a1e-aee8-4c8f467cd9b0.

21   Yasmine Ghania, "Record 417 COVID-19 Hospitalizations in Saskatchewan, 22 More Deaths Reported," *CBC News,* April 21, 2022, https://www.cbc.ca/news/canada/saskatchewan/record-417-covid-19-hospitalizations-in-saskatchewan-22-more-deaths-reported-1.6426687.

22   Adam Hunter, "Sask. Government Resists Opposition Calls for Daily COVID Reporting, Says Public Not Requesting It," *CBC News,* March 19, 2022, https://www.cbc.ca/news/canada/saskatchewan/sask-government-covid-1.6389813.

23   Shannon Gormley, "Why COVID-19 Spreads So Quickly Inside Dictatorships," *Maclean's,* March 6, 2020, https://www.macleans.ca/opinion/why-covid-19-spreads-so-quickly-inside-dictatorships/.

24   Tara J. Moriarty et al., *Excess All-Cause Mortality during the COVID-19 Epidemic in Canada* (Royal Society of Canada, June 29, 2021), https://rsc-src.ca/sites/default/files/EM%20PB_EN.pdf.

25   Alexander Quon, "Sask. Might Not Have Counted All COVID-19 Deaths, Excess Mortality Numbers Suggest," *CBC News,* May 18, 2022, https://www.cbc.ca/news/canada/saskatchewan/excess-mortality-sask-covid-1.6447074.

26   Adam Hunter, "Researcher Defends Work after Sask. Premier Calls COVID-19 Death Study 'Misinformation,'" *CBC News,* January 26, 2022, https://www.cbc.ca/news/canada/saskatchewan/sask-covid-deaths-uoft-1.6326802.

27   Moe, "Today, trucker rallies are being held at many locations across the country."

28   Zak Vescera, "COVID-19: Moe Scrapping Proof of Vaccination, Repeats Falsehoods on Vaccines," *Saskatoon StarPhoenix,* January 31, 2022, https://thestarphoenix.com/news/saskatchewan/covid-19-moe-scrapping-proof-of-vaccination-repeats-falsehoods-on-vaccines.

29   David N. Fisman, Afia Amoako, and Ashleigh R. Tuite, "Impact of Population Mixing between Vaccinated and Unvaccinated Subpopulations on Infectious Disease Dynamics: Implications for SARS-CoV-2 Transmission," *CMAJ* 194, 16 (2022): e573–e580, https://doi.org/10.1503/cmaj.212105.

30   Scott Moe (@PremierScottMoe), "Getting vaccinated is the best thing we can all do to protect ourselves and those around us and get life back to normal," Twitter, April 15, 2021, https://twitter.com/premierscottmoe/status/1382851936022450176.

31   Vescera, "COVID-19: Moe Scrapping Proof of Vaccination."

32   Mandryk, "Moe's Decision to Remove COVID-19 Restrictions Doesn't Add Up."

33   Andrew Caddell, "The MOU Says Everything You Need to Know about the Truckers Protest," *Hill Times*, February 2, 2022, https://www.hilltimes.com/story/2022/02/02/the-mou-says-everything-you-need-to-know-about-the-truckers-protest/270162/.

34   Yasmine Ghania, "Sask. Premier Scott Moe Criticized for Declining to Denounce Anti-Vaccine Mandate Protests," *CBC News*, February 10, 2022, https://www.cbc.ca/news/canada/saskatchewan/ndp-premier-scott-moe-anti-vaccine-mandate-protest-1.6346969.

35   Hunter, "How Sask. Premier Moe's Messaging on Unvaccinated People Has Shifted."

36   Moises Canales-Lavigne, "Saskatchewan Recorded Its Third-Highest Monthly COVID-19 Death Total in February," *Global News*, March 4, 2022, https://globalnews.ca/news/8659465/sask-covid-deaths-feb-2022/.

Waving Goodbye

1   Erin Griffith, "People Are Panic-Buying Meat, Toilet Paper ... and Pelotons?" *New York Times*, May 6, 2020, https://www.nytimes.com/2020/05/06/technology/peloton-boom-workout-virus.html.

2   Gus Carlson, "Peloton's Brand Crash Is a Symptom of Pandemic Fatigue, Not the Product's Fault," *Globe and Mail*, January 28, 2022, https://www.theglobeandmail.com/business/commentary/article-pelotons-brand-crash-is-a-symptom-of-pandemic-fatigue-not-the-products/.

3   Daniella Ponticelli, "'I Am Tired': A Leader in Sask. Pandemic Response Is Leaving the Health Authority," *CBC News*, February 18, 2022, https://www.cbc.ca/news/canada/saskatchewan/kevin-wasko-sha-pandemic-leader-leaves-1.6356933.

4   Laura Woodward, "Why a Doctor Who Helped Lead Saskatchewan's Pandemic Response Says He's Leaving the Province," *CTV News*, February 25, 2022, https://saskatoon.ctvnews.ca/why-a-doctor-who-helped-lead-saskatchewan-s-pandemic-response-says-he-s-leaving-the-province-1.5796464.

5   Ponticelli, "'I Am Tired.'"

6   Canadian Press, "Many Canadian Doctors Struggle with Burnout, Depression and Anxiety: Survey," *Toronto Star*, August 25, 2022, https://www.thestar.com/business/2022/08/25/many-canadian-doctors-struggle-with-burnout-depression-and-anxiety-survey.html.

7   Carly Lewis, "I've Only Been a Nurse for Eight Months. The Chaos Is Killing Me," *Maclean's*, August 4, 2022, https://www.macleans.ca/society/health/ive-only-been-a-nurse-for-eight-months-the-chaos-is-killing-me/.

8   Laura Woodward, "Sask. Health Authority Sees 4,000 Per Cent Increase in Staff Overtime during COVID-19 Pandemic," *CTV News*, May 25, 2021, https://saskatoon.ctvnews.ca/sask-health-authority-sees-4-000-per-cent-increase-in-staff-overtime-during-covid-19-pandemic-1.5442034.

9 Michelle McCarron et al., "Moral Injury within Canadian Frontline Healthcare Workers," Saskatchewan Health Authority, https://www.saskhealthauthority.ca/our-organization/our-direction/research/who-we-are/exciting-discoveries/moral-injury-within-canadian-frontline-healthcare-workers.

10 Saskatchewan Medical Association, "SMA Survey Reveals Impact of Pandemic on Saskatchewan's Physicians," news release, April 27, 2022, https://www.sma.sk.ca/?p=7374.

11 Kaylyn Whibbs, "More Than Half of Sask. Nurses Surveyed Are Considering Leaving the Profession: Union Poll," *CTV News*, April 5, 2022, https://regina.ctvnews.ca/more-than-half-of-sask-nurses-surveyed-are-considering-leaving-the-profession-union-poll-1.5849098.

12 Zak Vescera, "Sask. Doctors Are Tired, Demoralized and Considering Quitting: Survey," *Saskatoon StarPhoenix*, May 3, 2022, https://thestarphoenix.com/news/saskatchewan/sask-doctors-are-tired-demoralized-and-considering-quitting-survey.

13 Jeremy Simes, "Moe Stands by 'I Don't Care' Comment over Per Capita Emissions," *Regina Leader-Post*, April 11, 2022, https://leaderpost.com/news/saskatchewan/moe-stands-by-i-dont-care-comment-over-per-capita-emissions.

14 Rachel Sloane, "Resident of Camp Marjorie Dies following Overdose, Camp Leaders Say," *CBC News*, October 26, 2021, https://www.cbc.ca/news/canada/saskatchewan/first-fatal-overdose-camp-marjorie-1.6226276.

15 Connor O'Donovan, "At Least 9 Former Camp Hope Residents Dead of Overdose since Shut Down: Organizers," *Global News*, March 21, 2022, https://globalnews.ca/news/8698204/camp-hope-residents-overdose-deaths/.

16 For 2020 overdose deaths, see Thia James, "Saskatchewan May Suffer Up to 450 Fatal Drug Overdoses This Year," *Saskatoon StarPhoenix*, November 2, 2022, https://thestarphoenix.com/news/local-news/saskatchewan-may-suffer-up-to-450-fatal-drug-overdoses-this-year. For 2021 and 2022 deaths, see Larissa Kurz, "Sask. Reaches New Record for Overdoses in 2022," *Regina Leader-Post*, January 9, 2023, https://leaderpost.com/news/saskatchewan/sask-reaches-new-record-for-overdose-deaths-in-2022.

17 "About Us," Partners In Health Canada, https://pihcanada.org/about-us/.

18 Paul Farmer, *Pathologies of Power: Structural Violence and the Assault on Human Rights* (Berkeley: University of California Press, 2003), 26.

19 Albert Camus, *The Plague*, trans. Robin Buss (London: Penguin Books, 2001), 98.

Lessons for the Next Wave

1 For COVID deaths in Canada, see "COVID-19 Epidemiology Update: Key Updates," https://health-infobase.canada.ca/covid-19/. For COVID deaths in Saskatchewan, see Larissa Kurz, "Sask. COVID-19 Deaths Top 2021 Data, Expert Urges Caution over Holidays," *Regina Leader-Post*, December 22, 2022, https://leaderpost.com/news/sask-covid-19-deaths-top-2021-data-expert-urges-caution-over-holidays.

2 "Constitution," World Health Organization, https://www.who.int/about/governance/constitution.

3 Eeva Ollila, Fran Baum, and Sebastián Peña, "Introduction to Health in All Policies and the Analytical Framework of the Book," in *Health in All Policies: Seizing Opportunities, Implementing Policies*, ed. Kimmo Leppo et al. (Helsinki: Ministry of Social Affairs and Health, 2013), 3, http://www.euro.who.int/__data/assets/pdf_file/0007/188809/Health-in-All-Policies-final.pdf?ua=1.

4 Joe Hasell, "Which Countries Have Protected Both Health and the Economy in the Pandemic?" *Our World in Data*, September 1, 2020, https://ourworldindata.org/covid-health-economy.

5 Andrew Nikiforuk, "Canada Is One Big Pandemic Response Experiment. It Proves 'Zero COVID' Is Best," *The Tyee*, April 2, 2021, https://thetyee.ca/News/2021/04/02/Canada-One-Big-Pandemic-Response-Experiment-Zero-COVID/?fbclid=IwAR3TxSpDz9wW8ajU6RJb5N6045DU9BRNTrCyyY5KbmQ4QPSEhjTiS2SMyK4.

6 Steven Lewis, Nazeem Muhajarine, and Cory Neudorf, "Your Money or Your Life? Scott Moe's Tragic Miscalculation," *CBC News*, April 8, 2021, https://www.cbc.ca/news/canada/saskatchewan/opinion-lewis-muhajarine-neudorf-1.5978305.

7 Marek Kochańczyk and Tomasz Lipniacki, "Pareto-Based Evaluation of National Responses to COVID-19 Pandemic Shows That Saving Lives and Protecting Economy Are Non-Trade-Off Objectives," *Scientific Reports* 11, 2425 (2021), https://doi.org/10.1038/s41598-021-81869-2.

8 "A Remote Canadian Province Luxuriates in the Global Supply Crunch," *The Economist*, August 18, 2022, https://www.economist.com/the-americas/2022/08/18/a-remote-canadian-province-luxuriates-in-the-global-supply-crunch.

9 John Paul Tasker, "Vaccine Envy: Why Can't Canada Make COVID-19 Doses at Home?" *CBC News*, April 28, 2021, https://www.cbc.ca/news/politics/domestic-vaccine-manufacturing-canada-1.6004427.

10 #TransformSK, *The Upstream Economy: A Generational Dialogue for Transformative Change* (Regina: #TransformSK, 2019), https://saskchamber.com/isl/uploads/2019/04/TransformSK-Report.pdf.

11 #TransformSK, *The Upstream Economy*.

12 "The Care Economy Statement," Care Economy, https://thecareeconomy.ca/statement/.

13 Commission on Social Determinants of Health, *Closing the Gap in a Generation: Health Equity through Action on the Social Determinants of Health* (Geneva: World Health Organization, 2008), https://apps.who.int/iris/bitstream/handle/10665/43943/9789241563703_eng.pdf.

14 "Social Inequalities in COVID-19 Deaths in Canada," Government of Canada, August 26, 2022, https://health-infobase.canada.ca/covid-19/inequalities-deaths/.

15 Sabrina Jonas and Benjamin Shingler, "The Pandemic Exposed Montreal's Inequalities, and Residents Say It's Time to Tackle Root Causes," *CBC News*, November 3, 2021, https://www.cbc.ca/news/canada/montreal/covid-19-montreal-disparity-solutions-1.6232359.

16 "Why Have Some Places Suffered More Covid-19 Deaths Than Others?" *The Economist*, July 31, 2021, https://www.economist.com/finance-and-economics/2021/07/31/why-have-some-places-suffered-more-covid-19-deaths-than-others.

17 "Why Have Some Places Suffered."

18 Frank J. Elgar, Anna Stefaniak, and Michael J.A. Wohl, "The Trouble with Trust: Time-Series Analysis of Social Capital, Income Inequality, and COVID-19 Deaths in 84 Countries," *Social Science and Medicine* 263 (2020): 1–6, https://doi.org/10.1016/j.socscimed.2020.113365.

19 Richard G. Wilkinson and Kate Pickett, *The Spirit Level: Why Greater Equality Makes Societies Stronger* (New York: Bloomsbury, 2010).

20 Charlene Galarneau, "Getting King's Words Right," *Journal of Health Care for the Poor and Underserved* 29, 1 (2018): 5–8, https://muse.jhu.edu/article/686948/pdf.

21 Michael Marmot et al., *Build Back Fairer: The COVID-19 Marmot Review: The Pandemic, Socioeconomic and Health Inequalities in England* (London: Institute of Health Equity, 2020).

22 World Health Organization (@WHO), Twitter, February 15, 2020, https://twitter.com/WHO/status/1228683949796470784.

23 Bonnie Allen, "How a 36-Year-Old Yorkton Mother Died from COVID-19 at Home after Trying to 'Ride It Out,'" *CBC News*, November 19, 2021, https://www.cbc.ca/news/canada/saskatchewan/yorkton-mother-died-covid-1.6254486.

24 Stephen Maher, "Misinformation from the U.S. Is the Next Virus – and It's Spreading Fast," *Maclean's*, January 3, 2022, https://www.macleans.ca/society/health/misinformation-from-the-u-s-is-the-next-virus-and-its-spreading-fast/.

25 André Picard, "Lessons from Two Years of Pandemic Living," *Globe and Mail*, March 11, 2022, https://www.theglobeandmail.com/canada/article-lessons-from-two-years-of-pandemic-living/.

26 Will McLernon, "Sask. Health Authority Removes Online List of Family Doctors Accepting New Patients," *CBC News*, December 1, 2022, https://www.cbc.ca/news/canada/saskatchewan/health-authority-eliminates-online-database-doctors-accepting-new-patients-1.6670526.

27 Kathy Tomlinson and Grant Robertson, "Ottawa Had a Playbook for a Coronavirus-Like Pandemic 14 Years Ago. What Went Wrong?" *Globe and Mail*, April 9, 2020, https://www.theglobeandmail.com/canada/article-ottawa-had-a-playbook-for-a-coronavirus-like-pandemic-14-years-ago/.

28 Tomlinson and Robertson, "Ottawa Had a Playbook."

29 Geoff Leo, "Health Minister Reviewing Management of Canada's Emergency Stockpile," *CBC News*, April 15, 2020, https://www.cbc.ca/news/canada/saskatchewan/heath-minister-emergency-stockpile-1.5530081.

30 Murray Brewster, "Public Health Agency Was Unprepared for the Pandemic and 'Underestimated' the Danger, Auditor General Says," *CBC News*, March 25, 2021, https://www.cbc.ca/news/politics/auditor-general-pandemic-covid-phac-1.5963895.

31   Thilina Bandara, "Ontario Public Health Cuts Will Endanger the Public," *Conversation*, May 12, 2019, https://theconversation.com/ontario-public-health -cuts-will-endanger-the-public-116502.

32   Legislative Assembly of Saskatchewan, *Debates and Proceedings*, 28th Leg., 4th Sess. (March 17, 2020) (Scott Moe, Saskatchewan Party), https://docs.legassem-bly.sk.ca/legdocs/Legislative%20Assembly/Hansard/28L4S/200317Debates.pdf.

33   John Moraros, Mark Lemstra, and Chijioke Nwankwo, "Lean Interventions in Healthcare: Do They Actually Work? A Systematic Literature Review," *International Journal for Quality in Health Care* 28, 2 (2016): 150–65.

34   "Our Work," Remember Rebuild Saskatchewan, https://rememberrebuild.ca/.

35   "Remember Lives Not Numbers," Remember Rebuild Saskatchewan, https://rememberrebuild.ca/remember-lives-not-numbers/.

36   "Mortality Analyses," Coronavirus Resource Center, Johns Hopkins University and Medicine, https://coronavirus.jhu.edu/data/mortality.

37   Catherine Lévesque, "Theresa Tam Welcomes a Review of Canada's COVID Pandemic Response, Stresses Need for 'Humility,'" *National Post*, October 18, 2022, https://nationalpost.com/news/theresa-tam-welcomes-review-of-canadas -covid-pandemic-response-stresses-need-for-humility.

38   David Naylor et al., *Learning from SARS: Renewal of Public Health in Canada* (Ottawa: Health Canada, 2003), https://www.canada.ca/content/dam/phac -aspc/migration/phac-aspc/publicat/sars-sras/pdf/sars-e.pdf.

39   Tonda MacCharles, "Justin Trudeau Won't Commit, but a Top Health Adviser Says Canada Will Need an Inquiry into Its Pandemic Response," *Toronto Star*, May 16, 2021, https://www.thestar.com/politics/federal/2021/05/16/justin -trudeau-wont-commit-but-a-top-health-adviser-says-canada-will-need-an -inquiry-into-its-pandemic-response.html.

40   Richard Zussman, "B.C. to Review Pandemic Response, but Not Govern-ment or Public Health Decisions," *Global News*, March 16, 2022, https:// globalnews.ca/news/8688693/bc-pandemic-response-review/.

41   Adam Hunter, "Sask. NDP Leader Calls for Public Inquiry into Province's COVID-19 Response," *CBC News*, March 3, 2021, https://www.cbc.ca/news/ canada/saskatchewan/sask-ndp-covid-inquiry-1.5935422.

42   Larissa Kurz, "Sask. Opposition Calling for Public Inquiry into the Gov-ernment's COVID Response," *SaskToday.ca*, December 8, 2021, https://www. sasktoday.ca/south/local-news/sask-opposition-calling-for-public-inquiry -into-governments-covid-response-4845234.

43   Russel Wangersky, "Wangersky: Inquiries Can Offer Lessons, Not Just Become the Blame Game," *Regina Leader-Post*, March 25, 2022, https://leaderpost.com/ opinion/columnists/inquiries-dont-have-to-be-the-blame-game.

44   Simon Little and John Hua, "Majority of Canadians Back Inquiries into National, Provincial Pandemic Responses: Poll," *Global News*, April 22, 2022, https://globalnews.ca/news/8779585/canadians-inquiries-national-provincial -pandemic-response-poll/.

45   Wangersky, "Wangersky: Inquiries."

46 Emily Oster, "Let's Declare a Pandemic Amnesty," *The Atlantic,* October 31, 2022, https://www.theatlantic.com/ideas/archive/2022/10/covid-response-forgiveness/671879/.

47 J.V. Lazarus et al., "A Multinational Delphi Consensus to End the COVID-19 Public Health Threat," *Nature* 611 (2022): 332–45, https://doi.org/10.1038/s41586-022-05398-2.

Index

Note: "(f)" after a page number indicates an illustration. CMHO stands for chief medical health officer; PPE stands for personal protective equipment; RM stands for Ryan Meili; SARM stands for Saskatchewan Association of Rural Municipalities; SHA stands for Saskatchewan Health Authority.

children: catching up by, 105–7; child welfare system, 61; as COVID orphans, 100; deaths, 104; hospitalizations, 104–5, 229; impact on, xii; learning gaps among, 105; mental health of, 99; politicization of health/well-being, 98; in poverty, 101; respiratory infections, 104; RM's press conference for, 40; vaccination of, 105, 106, 136–37, 179–81, 189. *See also* young people

Children's Health Coalition, 106

circuit-breakers, 85, 144–45

Clark, Charlie, 27

classrooms. *See* schools

Clearwater River Dene Nation, 55–56, 175

Closing the Gap, 72

Closing the Gap in a Generation (Commission on Social Determinants of Health), 220

Coe, Jeannie, 49, 50, 132

Coleman, Rob, 114(f)

College of Family Physicians of Canada (Saskatchewan Chapter), 86

College of Physicians and Surgeons of Saskatchewan, 6, 48, 86

Commission on Social Determinants of Health, *Closing the Gap in a Generation*, 220

Community Care Kitchen, 32

community transmission. *See* transmission

Connect, Contrast, Solve (CCS), 71

contact tracing, 48–49, 172; added capacity for, 229; in Atlantic Canada, 144; Delta variant and, 160; deployment of health care workers for, 168, 169; introduction of, 110; during second wave, 84, 86

Co-operative Commonwealth Federation (CCF), 5–6, 67–68

Core Neighbourhood testing site, 48

Cornerstone School Division, 105–6

COVID-19: disruption of, 215; downplaying, 224; history of, 18–19;

inequality in, 220–21; as instructive, 215; lessons from, 13, 215–33; as life-changing, 232–33; living with, 195; national responses to, 231; as polycrisis, 12; post-pandemic reviews, 231–32; as revealing vs. causing problems, 12; scientific understanding of, 223–24

Cowessess First Nation, 112

cross-party collaboration, 24, 27–28, 29, 46–47, 226–27

Daly, Tamara, 123

death rates, xiv; during first wave, 15, 67, 110; during second wave, 79, 84, 116; during third wave, 125, 143; during fourth wave, 153, 158, 160, 170, 174, 175; during fifth wave, 185; in 2022 vs. 2020–21, 215; in Alberta, 109; in Atlantic Canada, 144, 145; in Canada, 12; and economy, 174; equality and, 221; in Japan, 53; in long-term care, 121; misinformation and, 222; modelling, 39; in New Zealand, 53; in North, 56; Omicron and, 191, 192, 195, 196, 200, 202; from overdosing, 210–11; poverty and, 220, 221; reporting of, 195; in Saskatchewan, 12, 109; as surpassing SARS, 21; in United States, 231

deaths: ageism and, 109; of celebrities, 36; of children, 104; first Canadian, 23; Grove as first Saskatchewan, 43; of homeless people, 165, 209; inequality and, 220; Lighthouse residents and, 50; locations of, 44; in long-term-care homes, 108, 109, 110, 114, 115, 116, 119, 121; numbers of excess, 197; from overdose, 73, 165; reporting of, 225; of seniors, 109; unreported, 12; of unvaccinated people, 4, 170; of vulnerable people, 109; of young people, 4

Degenstein, Paul, 71

Delta variant, 3–5, 157, 160, 188, 190, 191, 195–96

democracy, 212–13; disinformation and, 223; information and, 196; transparency and, 226

Devine, Grant, 20, 68

Dickson, Gerri, 127

Dickson, Graham, 167–69

Dickson, Helen (story), 167–69, 189, 230

Dickson, Murray, 127

Dix, Adrian, 110

doctors. *See* physicians

Doctors for Justice in Long-Term Care, 88

Donna (story), 69

Dosani, Naheed, 50

Douglas, Tommy, 5–6, 67–68, 211

drugs, 164, 165, 209–10. *See also* addictions

Duclos, Jean-Yves, 183, 231

Duncan, Dustin, 101, 106, 113, 179, 180

Durocher, Tristen, 57–58, 59–62, 63, 72, 189

Ebola, 137

economy: boom-and-bust cycles of, 219; caregivers and, 219–20; circuit breakers and, 144–45; death rates and, 174; elimination approach and, 218; health and, 216, 218–20; Indigenous peoples and, 72; public health and, 145; schools and, 107; wage levels and, 151

Eddie (Lighthouse resident), 133

education: funding, 102; Indigenous peoples and, 62, 63, 219; online learning, 37; reading levels, 73; Sarah story, 69; as social determinant of health, 106–7. *See also* schools; teachers

elderly people. *See* seniors

election, Saskatchewan 2020, 20–21, 25–26, 65–66, 67–76; election day, 74–75; incumbent governments returning, 75; leaders' debate, 70–74; modelling and, 84; results, 75–76;

social distancing during, 26, 65–66, 68–69

election, Unites States 2020, 44

elimination approach, 53–54, 218

employment: export of jobs, 69; during first wave, 33; Paul story, 69; precariousness of, 149–50; rebound, 145; school closures, and women's, 101; sick leave, 150; unemployment, 69, 149

endemic fatalism, 193

equality/equity, 63; and death rates, 221; and health, xii, 8, 220–21

essential workers, 34

ethical triage, 157, 158, 171, 207

evidence-based responses, 190, 193, 199, 223

Extendicare, 108, 110, 112, 113–20, 121, 122

falsehoods. *See* misinformation

Farmer, Paul, 109, 111, 212–13; *Pathologies of Power*, 213

Ferrier, Jeff, 71

Fiddler-Potter, Merelda, 72

fifth wave: case counts, 185; death rates, 185; gathering limits during, 189–90; hospitalizations during, 174; public health measures during, 186

first wave: case counts, 15, 67; common experiences during, 35; death rates, 15, 67; isolation, 31–32; kindness during, 32–33, 35; in long-term-care homes, 108, 110; perception of time during, 31; public health measures, 16; in Saskatchewan vs. Ontario and Quebec, 66; in Saskatchewan vs. rest of Canada, 39; spring 2020, 35–39, 40–41; state of emergency, 20; timeline, 17, 21–22, 28

Fitzgerald, Janice, 180

flattening the curve, 23, 52, 53, 55, 130

Floyd, George, 57

Fontaine, Tina, 61

Ford, Doug, 227

Fougere, Michael, 27

fourth wave: and Armed Forces medical staff, 3; blaming of hard-hit communities/North for, 57; blaming of unvaccinated for, 188; case counts, 153, 158, 171, 172; contact tracing during, 160; death rates, 153, 158, 160, 170, 174, 175; health care crisis during, 173–74; hospitalizations during, 172, 174; lack of access to essential care during, 169–70; masks/masking during, 173; medical officers of health speaking out during, 87; modelling of, 159–60; public call for opposition action, 158–59; public health measures, 154; role of CMHO and, 89; SHA vs. government in, 182; testing during, 160; unvaccinated people and, 172; vaccination during, 135, 172; vaccine-only strategy during, 171

Fraser, Heather, 71

freedom convoy. *See* protests

Friesen, Mark, 174, 189

Froh, John, 157–58

frontline workers: government slowness to act and, 38; in long-term-care homes, 111; Matthew Cardinal story, 147–49; minimum wage, 55; Syed story, 150; triaging decisions, 95; vaccination of, 148

Gallays, Jennifer, 102, 103, 105, 106

Gardner, Dan, 192

gathering restrictions, 28, 29, 72, 126, 145, 146, 177; during second wave, 84; during fourth wave, 175; during fifth wave, 189–90, 194; household bubbles, 39, 126, 146. *See also* social distancing

Gormley, Shannon, 196

Grange, Adriana, 106

Grebinski, Leisha, 174–75

Grimes, Ruth, 101, 104

Grove, Alice (story), 42–44, 230

Grove, Bruce, 42

H1N1 pandemic, xii, 18, 20, 26

Hadjistavropoulos, Thomas, 111

Hajdu, Patty, 21, 156, 227

Halkett, Richard, 98

"The Hammer and the Dance" (Pueyo), 53

harm reduction. *See* addictions

Harpauer, Donna, 67

Harrison, Jeremy, 25, 29

Harvey, Kaitlyn, 208

health: and economy, 216, 218–20; equality/equity and, xii, 8, 220–21; importance of, 11; Indigenous peoples and, 219; politics and, 10; poverty and, 8; and societal success, 216–17; vulnerable people and, 221

Health Canada, 220

health care workers: burnout, xiii, 106, 207–8; deployment for testing/tracing, 168, 169; exhaustion of, 194; hours of work, 206–7; impact on, xiii; mandatory vaccination of, 160; and moral injury, xiv; numbers of, 229; speaking out during second wave, 86–87; vaccination, 131–32

health care/health care systems, 70; access to, 64; capacity in, 229–30; crisis in, xii, 173–74, 183–84, 228; impact on, xiv, 95, 227; "Lean" program, 228; long-term care integration into, 123; national, 183–84; need for care vs. ability to pay in, 184; pandemic planning and, 26; private vs. public, 228; redlining of, 228; robust/resilient, 227–30; universal, xii; user-pay scheme, 69

Health in All Policies, 217

health leaders. *See* medical health officers (MHOs)

A Healthy Society (Meili), 9, 10

Henry, Bonnie, 33, 88

Hicks, Jack, 58

Higgs, Blaine, 27

Hindley, Everett, 116

Hinshaw, Deena, 33

200; and RM's last legislature appearance, 211–12; school closure and, 100; during spring 2020, 36, 37, 38–39; in Walking With Our Angels, 59–60

Meili, Augustin (Gus), 141(f); contracts COVID-19, 200–2; during election campaign, 70; mask-wearing, 200; and RM's last legislature appearance, 211–12; during spring 2020, 36, 37

Meili, Jim, 6–7, 22, 36, 211

Meili, Lea, 110, 140, 141–42

Meili, Miles, 6–7

Meili, Ryan: burnout, 204–5; contracts COVID-19, 202; early life and education, 6–7, 22; and election, 65–66, 67–77; as family doctor vs. politician, 6, 9, 65; family medical practice, 8; giving vaccines at Merlis Belsher Place, 5–6; *A Healthy Society*, 9, 10; at Lighthouse, 48, 49, 50–51; at medical school, 7–8; and Moose Jaw Extendicare, 110; in Mozambique, 127–28; participation in Walking With Our Angels, 59–60; political career, 8–9; press conference for children, 40; resignation as NDP leader, 203–4, 205, 211–12; returns to medical practice, 9, 40, 48, 90–91; SARM address, 22–23, 24; during spring 2020, 35–39; responds to overdose, 209–11; vaccination, 129–30

Meili, Wally, 139, 140–42, 143–44, 176–77

mental health/illness, 62, 63–64, 69, 73, 99, 181–82, 207

Merasty, Chris, 59–61

Mercredi, Jason, 164–65

Merlis Belsher Place, 5–6, 132

Merriman, Paul, 83, 134, 158, 159, 180

Michael Garron Hospital, 177

minimum wage. *See under* wages

Ministry of Health: and excess deaths, 197; and Parkside Extendicare outbreak, 116; SHA relationship with, 182

misinformation, xii, 44, 197–99, 222–23; anti-vaccine, 46; complex information and, 223; factual information vs., 190; impact of, xii; information sharing vs., 226; limiting information and, 44; and vaccine hesitancy, 190. *See also* information sharing

mitigation strategy, 54, 144, 170–71, 224

Mitsuing, Ronald, 58

modelling, 39–40; case counts, 39; death rates, 39; Delta variant, 157–58; fourth wave, 159–60; information sharing regarding, 224; and masking, 171–72; Omicron, 191; and provincial election, 84; second wave, 83–84

Moderna vaccine, 130

Moe, Scott: and anti-vaccine movements, 172; blaming of northern/remote communities, 57, 172; and Buffalo Party, 77, 198; on carbon emissions, 208; during Delta wave, 188; displays of emotion, 143; and election, 20–21, 25, 71–74; on flattening curve, 52, 55; during fourth wave, 88, 160, 171, 174–75, 178–79; and freedom convoy, 187–88, 198–99; on government response to COVID, 44; and Great Saskatchewan Summer (2021), 156, 174–75; Grimes's letter regarding protection of children, 101; and Kenney, 156, 158; last regular public briefing, 155; on long-term care, 110; and masks/masking, 46, 72, 194; Masri on, 87; on medical community advocacy, 88; medical health officers' letters to, 178–79; misinformation from, 197–98; and Ness, 189; during Omicron wave, 188, 189–90, 191; and pandemic fatigue, 191–92; prolongation of outbreaks, 145; and proof-of-vaccination policy, 188, 199; and Regina ICU visit, 144–45; Re-Open Saskatchewan plan, 52,

54–55; and Re-Opening Roadmap, 134, 135, 155–56; and restrictions, 72, 146, 155–56, 160, 171, 188, 193–94, 199; RM on debating with, 208; on Royal Society of Canada study on excess deaths, 197; during second wave, 66; and Shahab, 89, 155, 194; on shutdowns, 77; and suicide prevention, 72; and summer 2021, 157, 158; testing positive, 193–94; and Trudeau, 66, 158, 172; and Unified Grassroots, 189–90; and unvaccinated people, 172–73, 188; on vaccination, 188, 198; and Wascana Park protest site, 61. *See also* Saskatchewan Party

Moms Stop the Harm, 73, 210

Moore, Joan, 114(f)

Moore, Pam, 114(f)

moral distress, 207

moral injury, xiv, 207, 208

Morgan, Don, 20

Moriarty, Tara, 12, 197

Morrow, Kendra, 56–57

Mowat, Vicki, 19, 26, 135

Muhajarine, Nazeem, 20, 87, 135, 146, 218

National Advisory Committee on Immunization, 164

National Institute on Ageing, 137; *Pandemic Perspectives on Long-Term Care*, 122

Naylor, David, 231–32

Neglected No More (Picard), 122

Ness, Nadine, 189

Neudorf, Cory, 87, 157, 160, 171, 173, 178–79, 218

New Brunswick: opposition leaders included in planning, 27; response to COVID, 27; return of incumbent government in, 75

New Democratic Party (NDP): during 2020 Saskatchewan election, 67–72; back-to-school plan, 102–3; convention, 181–82; fourth wave and call for action to, 158–59; leadership, 203–4, 208; People First campaign slogan, 69–70; People-First Recovery plan, 67; RM stepping down as leader, 203–4; Saskatchewan Party branding of, 68; during spring 2020, 37–38. *See also* election, Saskatchewan 2020; legislature; Meili, Ryan

New Zealand: death rates in, 53; government intervention in, 86; restrictions in, 53–54; return of incumbent government in, 75

Newfoundland and Labrador: all-party committee, 27; children's vaccination in, 180–81; public health nursing system in, 181

North, the: COVID-19 in, 55–57; vaccination rates in, 172

Notley, Rachel, 66

Nova Scotia: circuit breaker lockdown in, 144–45; informal caregiver compensation in, 124

nurses, 206–7; Brenda story, 69. *See also* health care workers

Nyee, Justin, 58

Oberik, Dallas (story), 169

Okeeweehow, Sharon, 70(f)

Olszynski, Paul, 87, 127–28

Omicron variant, 149, 188, 189–96, 198, 200, 202, 225

155 Collective, 56, 57

Ontario: Doctors for Justice in Long-Term care, 88; export of ICU patients to, xiv, 158, 171, 175, 177; long-term-care homes in, 108, 114; military use in, 54; public health cuts, 227; social housing, 47; state of emergency, 29; support payments, 55

Ontario Principals' Council, 106

Ontario Science Table, 120

Operation Warp Speed, 130

opposition: cross-party collaboration and, 226–27; as toxic to soul, 159. *See also* New Democratic Party (NDP)

organ donations/transplants, 167, 169;
Bailey story, 165, 230
Organisation for Economic Co-
operation and Development
(OECD) countries: deaths, 53; long-
term-care deaths in, 108
Ottawa: freedom convoy at, 187–88,
198–99; protests in, xiii

Palangi, Monga (story), 91, 93–95, 230
Palangi, Sherstin, 93, 95
Palliative Education and Care for the
Homeless (PEACH), 50
pandemic fatigue, 191–92
*Pandemic Perspectives on Long-Term
Care* (National Institute on Ageing
and Canadian Medical Association),
122
pandemics: defined, 23; post-pandemic
reviews, 231–32
Partners In Health (PIH), 212–13
Pathologies of Power (Farmer), 213
Paul (story), 69
Peiris, Sarath, 88–89, 90
People-First Recovery plan (NDP), 67
People's Party of Canada (PPC), 174,
189
Pepsi Park, 209–11
personal protective equipment (PPE),
45, 92, 119
Pfizer-BioNTech COVID-19 vaccine,
128, 130, 189
Pharmacare, 228
Pharmacy Association of Saskatchewan, 86
physical distancing. *See* social
distancing
Physician Town Halls, 146, 158, 175, 182
physicians: advocacy by, xii–xiii, 87–
88; burnout, 95, 206; contracting
COVID, 93–95; and COVID-19,
85–96; letters, 85–86, 189; mental
health, 207; and moral injury, xiv;
and Omicron, 194; shortage, 228;
visits to long-term care homes,
118–19

Picard, André, 108–9, 123, 193, 224, 225;
Neglected No More, 122
Pickett, Kate, *The Spirit Level*, 221
Pillars for Life, 58, 61
Pine Grove Correctional Centre, 164
Pioneer Village home, 115
The Plague (Camus), 3, 15, 36, 79, 125,
153, 185, 213
pneumonia, 18; Palangi story, 93–95
Poilievre, Pierre, 198
politics: and health, 10; medicine and,
8–9; science and, xiii–xiv; social
determinants of health and, 9; well-
being and, 4–5
populism, 198
poverty, 62; children living in, 101; and
death rates, 220, 221; and health, 8;
impact on people living in, 11; physicians and, 213. *See also* homeless
people /homelessness; vulnerable
people
Prairie Harm Reduction, 164
Prince Albert Grand Council, 83
Prince Edward Island, opposition
leaders included in planning, 27
Prine, John, 36
prisons, 160–64, 221; Cory Cardinal
story, 160–65; Squirrel story, 164
Pro Bono Law group, 161
Protect Our Province Alberta, 88
protests, xiii, 57, 59–61, 89, 187–88, 198–99
Provincial Emergency Operations
Centre, 182
public good, 34–35
public health: added capacity in, 229–
30; cuts to, xii, 20, 227; and economy,
145; exhaustion of appetite for campaigns, 137; funding, xii, 227; misinformation and, 223; officials, 33–34;
prevention in, 83–84; spending, 20
Public Health Agency of Canada,
231–32
public health measures: during first
wave, 16, 39; during second wave,
80; during third wave, 126; during
fourth wave, 154, 155–56; during fifth

wave, 186; on gatherings, 28, 29, 72, 126, 145, 177; and individual freedoms, 156; lifting/removal of, 146, 154, 155–56, 157–58, 186, 194, 199; in medical health officers' letter to Moe, 178–79; Moe and, 193–94; in New Zealand, 53–54; Omicron and, 194–95; and prevention of infection, 178; travel, 22, 23, 28, 126, 144; vaccination and, 134, 156

Public Health Montreal, 220

public health officials: government vs., 146; politicians hiding behind, 90

Pueyo, Tomas, "The Hammer and the Dance," 53

Quebec: long-term care in, 114; military use in, 54; posthumous testing in, 197; social housing in, 47

Quinn, Terry, 187–88

racism, 63

Rankin, Iain, 145

Raphael, Dennis, 10, 11

REACH, 6, 132

Regina Fire Department, 115

Regina General Hospital, 139, 148; ICU, 143–44

Regina Pasqua hospital, 112

Reid, Graham, 68

Reiter, Jim, 19, 20

"Remember Lives Not Numbers," 230–31

"Remember Rebuild Saskatchewan," 230

renewable energy, 69, 70

Re-Open Saskatchewan plan, 52, 54–55

Re-Opening Roadmap, 134

residential schools, 62, 63

restrictions. *See* public health measures

Revera Inc., 122

Reverse School Bus project, 32

right, political: move to, in Saskatchewan, 68; and political vs. moral, 196; Saskatchewan Party and, 77

"Risk of Fall Surge," 157–58

Romanow, Roy, 10, 68, 211

Roth, Ken (story), 175–76, 177–78, 230

Roth, Lorraine, 175, 176

Royal College of Physicians and Surgeons of Canada, 87

Royal Society of Canada, 197

Royal University Hospital (RUH), 6, 91–92, 131(f), 229

safe consumption sites. *See* addictions; drugs

Safe Schools Saskatchewan, 102, 103

Sarah (story), 69

Sarauer, Nicole, 161

SARS epidemic, xii, 18, 21, 227, 231–32

SARS-CoV-2, 18, 21, 45, 92, 94, 103

Sasakamoose, Fred (story), 81–83, 95, 230; *Call Me Indian*, 83

Sasakamoose, Leo, 82

Sasakamoose, Loretta, 81, 82

Sasakamoose, Neil, 81–83, 157

Sasakamoose, Peter, 82

Saskatchewan Association of Rural Municipalities (SARM), 22–23, 24, 25

Saskatchewan College of Pharmacy Professionals, 86

Saskatchewan Health Authority (SHA), 21; calls on identified positives, 222; Executive Leadership Team, 183, 205; modelling regarding cases/deaths, 39; and Parkside Extendicare outbreak, 116, 118, 120, 121; Physician Town Halls, 146, 158, 175, 182; and prison vaccine rollouts, 164; and Regina ICU visits, 144; relationship with Ministry of Health, 182–83; and updates of projections, 84; and vaccinations, 131–32; Wilson on, 183

Saskatchewan Medical Association, 86, 179; physician mental health survey, 207

Saskatchewan Party: branding of NDP, 68; and Buffalo Party, 198; dominance of, 67; and election

2020, 20–21; and living with COVID, 195; and long-term care, 111, 121; origins, 20; pandemic revealing quality of government, 203; prolongation of outbreaks, 145; and schools, 103; and snap election, 20–21; and suicide prevention, 58–59, 61–62; and Unified Grassroots, 189; and vaccination, 135, 180, 181; and vulnerable people, 47. *See also* election, Saskatchewan 2020; legislature; Moe, Scott

Saskatchewan Population Health and Evaluation Research Unit (SPHERU), 134–35

Saskatchewan Registered Nurses' Association, 86

Saskatchewan Teachers' Federation, 97, 179

Saskatchewan Union of Nurses, 86, 88, 207

Saskatoon Inter-Agency Response, 47–48

Saskatoon Provincial Correctional Center, 161, 163

Saskatoon Public Schools, 106

Saskatoon Tribal Council, 83

Sawatsky, Leah, 131

Scheer, Andrew, 71

schools: classroom sizes, 69, 70, 72, 73, 102, 105; closures, 37, 98–101; and economy, 107; masks/masking in, 84, 103, 106; medical health officers and, 179; in Mozambique, 128; NDP back-to-school plan, 102–3; parental notification when children testing positive, 194–95; proof of vaccination in, 179; removal of restrictions, 194–95; residential schools, 62, 63; second wave outbreaks in, 104; social distancing in, 97, 103; vaccinations in, 180; ventilation, 102; viral spread in, and community transmission, 100–1. *See also* education; teachers

science, politics and, xiii–xiv

second wave: case counts, 79, 84, 85, 96, 104; death rates, 79, 84, 116; gathering limits during, 84; hospitalizations during, 84, 85; masks/masking during, 84; modelling of, 83–84; Moe's overconfidence regarding, 66; public health measures during, 80; school closures, 98–101; school outbreaks, 104; testing during, 84, 86; tracing during, 84, 86; vaccination during, 131, 135

self-isolation. *See* isolation

seniors: Cath story, 69; deaths of, 109; elder care, 108–9; home care, 69, 111–12; hospitalization of, 112–13; isolation of, 143; neglect of, 109, 111, 122; non-institutional care for, 122; vaccination of, 129, 132. *See also* long-term care (LTC)

Shahab, Izn, 19

Shahab, Qudrut Ullah, *Shahab Nama*, 34

Shahab, Saqib: about, 19, 33–34; breaking down in tears, 3–5, 175; as chief health medical officer, 88–90; freedom rally outside legislature on, 89; and #GreatSKSummer, 156; Grimes's letter to, 101; on mask use/discretionary contact, 194; on MHOs' stopgap measures, 179; and Moe, 89, 155, 194; picketing outside home, 89; press conference on vaccinations, 134; and protection of children, 101; and provincial health order during fourth wave, 179; on race between vaccine and variant, 146; RM and, 19; role, 182; warnings regarding fourth wave, 172

Sharon (story), 69

Shaw, Susan, 100, 147, 148, 175

Singh, Jagmeet, 71

Smart, Katharine, 173–74, 183

Smith, Danielle, 189, 198

social democracy. *See* democracy

social determinants of health, 7–8, 9, 10, 36–37, 69–70, 106–7, 217

Warner, Michael, 177
Wascana Park, 59, 60–61
Wasko, Kevin, 175, 205–6
waves of COVID, 52–53. *See also individual waves, and names of variants*
Weins, Laura, 167–69
Welyki, Gloria, 128–29
Welyki, Wally, 129
West Side Community Clinic, 6, 8, 49
White-Crummey, Arthur, 66, 83
Widdowson, Eleanor, 42–44
Wilkinson, Andrew, 71
Wilkinson, Richard, *The Spirit Level*, 221

Wilson, Raynelle, 183
Wingerter, Jacelyn, 206
working from home, 145, 149
World Health Organization (WHO), 21, 23, 163
Wyant, Gord, 103

young people: deaths of, 4; and hopelessness, 63; isolation of, 143; suicide among, 57–58. *See also* children

Zambory, Tracy, 88, 194

About the Author

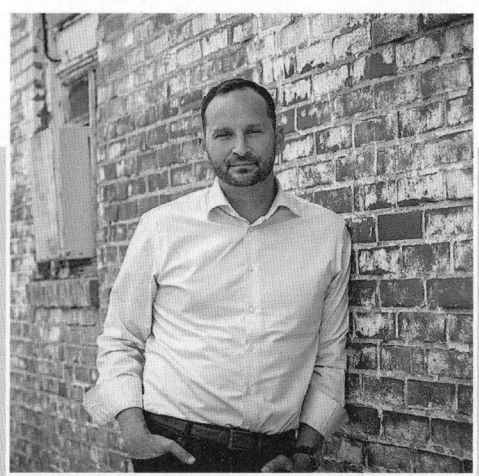

JOSHUA BERSON

RYAN MEILI is a family physician who focuses on health equity and social justice.

He is the author of *A Healthy Society: How a Focus on Health Can Revive Canadian Democracy*. He has practised family medicine in rural and Northern Saskatchewan, as well as in Saskatoon and rural Mozambique.

In 2017, Ryan Meili was elected as Member of Saskatchewan's Legislative Assembly for Saskatoon Meewasin, going on to serve as leader of the Saskatchewan New Democratic Party and leader of the official opposition in Saskatchewan from 2018 to 2022.

He lives in Saskatoon with his wife, Mahli Brindamour, and their two sons, Abe and Gus.

Printed and bound in Canada by Friesens
Set in Calibri and Sabon by Artegraphica Design Co. Ltd.
Substantive editor: Lesley Erickson
Copy editor: Francis Chow
Proofreader: Judith Earnshaw
Indexer: Noeline Bridge
Cover designer: Michel Vrana